LOOK BETTER, FEEL BETTER

LOOK BETTER,
FEEL BETTER

*The world-renowned Mensendieck System of
Functional Movements—for a youthful body
and vibrant health*

by BESS M. MENSENDIECK, M.D.

Foreword by Paul B. Magnuson, M.D.

Chairman, President's Committee on the Health Needs of the Nation

ILLUSTRATED

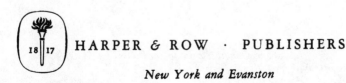

HARPER & ROW · PUBLISHERS

New York and Evanston

DEDICATION

To Annemarie Meusser, my alter
ego, in her idealistic conception and
interpretation of my work

APPRECIATION

I wish to express my sincere thanks to Amy Meusser for her unfailing co-operation.

To Dr. L. Larry Leonard in appreciation of his practical assistance in the preparation of this book. Without his untiring efforts this volume would still be unpublished.

To Mogens Hoff for his fine illustrations and for his patient efforts to present my conception of functional body movements.

To Harper & Brothers for their readiness to see the scope of my work and their co-operation in bringing the Mensendieck System of Body Education to the reading public.

CONTENTS

vii

CONTENTS

viii

CONTENTS

x

FOREWORD

The Mensendieck System has been of interest to me for many years in work in orthopedic surgery. The knowledge of anatomy and the mechanics of the body displayed by Dr. Mensendieck in setting up her system of exercises, and teaching the reason for these exercises to her students, has been extremely successful.

The System, if carried out and conscientiously followed by students and patients of those students, has given remarkable success in the treatment of faulty posture and early scoliosis (curvature of the spine). In these days of early exercise after surgery, and treatment of cardiac cases and neurologic cases by exercises, Dr. Mensendieck was far in advance of her time when she designed her system and began teaching it.

I can heartily endorse the exercises as having worked great good for many of my patients.

PAUL B. MAGNUSON, M.D.
Chairman, President's Committee
on the Health Needs of the Nation

Part I

THE KEY TO SHAPING
YOUR BODY

1.

BECOME THE SCULPTOR
OF YOUR BODY

You can now, in a sense, become a sculptor of your body, helping to shape its limbs and torso almost as though you were working with clay or marble. For within the given proportions of your bone structure, you—all men and women—have considerable choice in the lines your body will assume. Thus you can allow your body, through neglect, to sag, bulge and spread. Or you can so mold your figure as to bring it added grace and vigor.

This can be done because the outlines of the body depend upon the muscles which clothe the framework of bone. A heavy ankle, a bulging abdomen, a double chin—all of these reflect a poor condition of the muscles involved. Therefore, improve the condition of the muscles and the outline of the body becomes slender, the limbs taper gently, the waistline and chest become better proportioned. When muscles are in natural "tonic condition," the body is drawn tall and erect, and the head is held high, thereby reducing bulges and smoothing the facial and neck outlines.

With this, you will be adding vitality and strength to the body, thereby guarding it against aches and pains that may result from inadequately developed muscles. And you will also be protecting it against certain weaknesses of advancing age. For the means you use to sculpture the body are also the means to preserve its vitality throughout life.

In Search of a Method

The way to sculpture your body is comparatively simple, although it is built upon the scientific principles of anatomy, physics and body mechanics. We are presenting the method to you in a manner that will take but little time from your busy day. But to perfect this method, decades of patient scientific study, research and experimentation were necessary.

The work of many scientists contributed to the foundation upon which the Mensendieck System of Functional Movement is built. The first spark for the System itself, however, was *curiosity* aroused in a nonscientific setting, a Parisian academy of sculpturing where I was a student. This was curiosity concerning the differences in the shapes of people. If some models could have the beautiful lines of masterful Greek statues why couldn't others? To be sure, not everyone could be a Venus or an Adonis, but it seemed that many did not develop the full potentialities of their bodies.

4

Many of the models, I felt, could have had beautiful bodies, but were satisfied with less. A thigh was too heavy, or an arm puffy and crooked at the elbow joint, or badly held shoulders narrowed the chest. As the models took their poses some moved unevenly, arms and legs jerking as though a motor controlled them, jamming suddenly and starting abruptly again.

The professor at the academy in Paris, seeing my difficulty in shaping clay to conform to the live models, remarked with a smile one day, "You should become a sculptor in flesh and not in clay." He proved to be right. Sculpture in flesh was the answer for me.

The sciences pointed the way. While I was studying at the Medical College in Paris, the professors referred frequently to the great work of the mid-nineteenth century scientist, C. B. Duchenne. His research fanned the sparks of my curiosity into flames of hope that a method could be found to shape the human body.

Duchenne swept away the doubts concerning the function of muscles in the body by identifying the specific roles of many of them. Prior to that time, the study of anatomy had revealed the structure of muscle, but no one had proved what function each muscle performed. In his experiments, Duchenne used electric currents. For example, he applied a current to the nerve of the muscle that extends from the tip of the shoulder to the upper arm. The arm moved forward and upward. Thus, the electric current, via the proper nerve, directly stimulated the muscle to action.

Nonetheless, many questions were left unanswered. If an electric current stimulated the muscle into action, could not the brain do as much? Could not the will power of the individual be used to stimulate specific, neglected muscles? If will power were exerted and the muscle brought into use, what influence would this have upon the muscle shape?

From all sides came the answers and patient work began. People were hired to serve as "models." They were of various ages. Day after day the muscles that Duchenne had moved so readily with electricity were coaxed into action *consciously*. Again and again we had to say, "Think! Consciously use the muscle at the shoulder tip in front—the Front Deltoid—and with it raise the arm forward and upward." Gradually, the model transferred her thoughts correctly from her hand to her arm-raising muscles, the Deltoid. Thereafter when she wished to raise her arm, her thoughts automatically went to the shoulder-arm muscle.

With adequate muscle movement, the lines of the shoulder began to change, and the contours of the arm became more shapely. We worked similarly with other muscle groups and with other models. After about eight months of experimentation this work was reviewed by members of the medical faculty.

So impressed were they with the results that they urged that the experiments be continued.

Gradually, a workable method was developed and became known as the Mensendieck System. To the science of muscle function now was added the technique for teaching muscle control to others. This ultimately took the form of Movement Schemes, many of which are presented in this book. Then came the first phase in the application of the System. Working closely with physicians and hospitals, we sought to restore lost muscle function of those suffering disability after operations, from advanced age or because of paralysis. There followed lectures in many European cities.

Ultimately came the need to train "teachers" of the Mensendieck System so that all who wished to apply it in the improvement of their bodies could be shown the way. Through the issuance of certificates it was assured that only those who were qualified in the application of the Mensendieck principles could teach the Mensendieck System. Thus Mensendieck Institutes were founded on three continents, most numerously in Scandinavia and Germany.

The Mensendieck System is based upon the scientific fact that along with food and oxygen, the body needs *movement* to sustain its vitality and health, and also to preserve its natural graceful lines. Not just walking, sports and exercise, but proper movement according to the laws of body mechanics and

7

muscle function. How you move the parts of your body is important, crucially important.

Examine Your Movements

The way you are using your body will be partly revealed in the answers you give to these questions:

1. How do you get out of a chair?
   a) Pull myself up by the chair arms.
   b) Support myself by placing my hands on my thighs.
   c) Rise without support of hands.

2. When you bend is your abdomen
   a) Relaxed?
   b) Allowed to bulge loosely?
   c) Drawn in?

3. Do you bend your body sideways in the course of the day?
   a) Frequently.
   b) Occasionally.
   c) Seldom.

4. When you sit do you
   a) Shift your trunk to one side?
   b) Distribute weight evenly on sitting bones?
   c) Slump back in chair?

5. While standing or walking, are your buttock muscles
   a) Held tight?
   b) Kept relaxed, allowed to be soft and loose?

These answers indicate you are guarding the body through natural movements: 1*c*, 2*c*, 3*a* or *b*, 4*b*, 5*a*.

Functional Movement

The body requires movement, natural movement, in which muscles and joints are being used in accordance with the human anatomy and the science of body mechanics.

When you bend and raise your head, are you using the muscles in back of the neck? If not, you may develop a double chin or thick neck, for incorrect muscles are being used which draw the neckline out of shape.

When you raise your arm, are you conscious of the muscles near the end of the shoulder? If not, you will be inviting drooping shoulders rather than squared ones.

When you bend, do you draw in the long abdominal muscle? If not, your abdomen may bulge.

When you sit, do you use your sitting bone? If not, you are inviting backache.

Do you have heavy thighs? Then you are not using your thigh muscles in your daily movements.

When you stand or walk, where do you carry the weight of the body? If it is anywhere other than toward the ball of the foot, near the large toe, your body is out of line and you will see it in the shape of your ankles, calves, knees, thighs—right up to your shoulders.

When you stand up, do you shift the weight of the body from the sitting bones to the legs with the synchronized movement of your buttock muscles? If you pull yourself up by the arms of the chair, many parts of the body are being improperly used and you will see this in the shape of the buttocks and the thighs particularly.

So you see, if you are to sculpture your body, all that nature asks is that you regain the natural inclination for normal, functional movement.

When you sit down, stand up, reach, bend, etc., learn to do it in accordance with functional movements. If you don't, you are abusing muscles and joints, thereby depriving the body of the grace and vitality it should and readily could have.

Improper body use and *not* advancing age is the cause for sag, bulge and ache. Scientific analysis of the human anatomy confirms that nature has given us the means to maintain and preserve the looks of the body throughout life. Why not know and use these wonderful natural powers to full advantage?

Whatever the condition of the body, all can benefit. It is never too late. Just as a cut in the hand heals, and the fracture of a bone mends, so can parts of the body that sag or ache from lack of proper movement be restored.

You can do this by means of the basic Movement Schemes included in this book. These Movement Schemes are the culmination of more than forty years of research, experimentation and application. Thousands of people on three continents have benefited from them—from Hollywood stars and European royalty, to businessmen, factory workers and housewives.

You, too, can benefit. Through natural, functional movement:

> The abdomen can be flattened.
> The thighs remolded.
> Sagging breasts lifted.
> Ankles slenderized.
> A double chin smoothed.
> The buttocks shaped tightly.
> A weak back strengthened.

These changes can be brought about by the daily use of the Movement Schemes. Those who seek to maintain their muscles in tonic condition, thereby guarding the shape and health of the body, can use the Movement Schemes as self-instruction guides. You will learn from them how to use your body correctly in your daily activities, when you sit, bend, reach, walk or stand. If you are uncertain that you are reaching, in your daily activities, all the muscles that should be used regularly, you can be sure of reaching them by doing the appropriate Movement Schemes. For example, we seldom move our legs sideways in the course of the day. By means of Movement Scheme 26, page 199 you reach the exact muscles on which the shape of the outer thigh and the flexibility of the hip joint depend. We will point out in the instructions that accompany the Movement Schemes those which can best be used for this purpose.

For Women

The Mensendieck Movement Schemes provide an answer to women who have specific body problems:

How to improve a hipline or neckline.
What to do about crooked elbows and flabby upper arms.
How to prevent the breasts from sagging.
How to prevent household chores from taking a toll on attractive body outlines.

There is but one answer and it is the same for all of these problems. It is this: always make sure that the muscles around the area in question are in full tonic condition through correct movement.

This may sound oversimplified but let us examine

it more closely. Many women are distressed with their flabby buttock muscles, and their rounded abdominal line. When they are pregnant they worry whether they will carry the baby properly and safely. Yet the same muscles that shape the abdominal lines guard the baby.

We shall look at the details of this area of the body, the bony pelvis, later. It is enough to point out now that when these muscles are in tonic condition they help hold the bony pelvis in balance and thereby hold the abdominal organs in proper place. This affects the position of the womb, and facilitates carrying the baby correctly.

The problems of aching, tired feet, heavy ankles, swollen instep, flat feet, all of these common among women under ordinary circumstances, may become accentuated during pregnancy. Therefore, the corrective steps taken before pregnancy will become of added benefit during pregnancy.

Muscle control which is gained from the Movement Schemes preserves and improves the body's shape and, at the same time, guards the body's health. Take so simple, or seemingly simple, a matter as breathing. Correct use of the breathing muscles can affect the lines of the neck. Control of muscles, how to tense and relax them, will aid in the childbirth process itself. Similarly, proper care of the breast muscles affects the figure outline and the condition of the glands for breast-feeding.

Thus if women take steps to guard their figures, they also will be guarding their health. And the results will be apparent throughout life. The Movement Schemes in this book give the key to solving many difficulties and preventing others.

The experience of a woman of forty-three illustrates the beneficial results derived from the Movement Schemes. She came to the Mensendieck Institute because she was afraid her neckline would make her appear too old for a job she was applying for.

Apparently she had used her neck muscles improperly, for her neckline had started to become scrawny and hollows had appeared along the collar bone. Fortunately, the unattractive lines had not gone too far, and we could cope with them in the short time available.

Two Movement Schemes in particular reached the troubled area. One called Neck Forward Bend simply called for the head to be bent forward in a way to reach specific neck muscles. We give the full instructions in subsequent pages. This Movement she did before mirrors daily until she was so sure of the movement she could use it throughout the day whenever her activities required her to bend the head. A second Movement Scheme, Breast Muscle Control, merely called for her to raise her arms and bring them together in such a way as to reach the breast muscle. Since she seldom had the chance to use this movement in her activities she did this one daily as an exercise.

Before a month had passed the neckline had been sufficiently improved for her to go to the interview without fear of being thought too old. Soon afterward she received notice of her employment, she remarked that the Mensendieck System had transformed her whole life. But, more accurately, she had done the transforming with the help of nature's powers. What is more, she not only had transformed her neckline into a more graceful one, but also with the new movement habits she could keep it that way throughout life.

There are other examples we shall mention later; the dancer with the heavy thighs, the young mother seeking to reduce her outline after pregnancy, the woman troubled by heavy ankles. The answer for all of them, as for you, is found in functional movement.

For Men

Men, too, can now find the answers to many special bodily problems:

How to flatten the abdomen.
How to end the tired, aching feeling in the back.
How to overcome flat feet.
How to square the shoulders.

How to overcome nervous tension.

What to do about a double chin.

Men are prone to seek the answers to these problems in vigorous movements: the rowing machine, the hand ball or tennis court, gymnastic bars and dumbbells. Whatever contributions vigorous sports and exercise may make to the body—and we shall examine these later—they may not resolve problems such as these.

On the contrary, they may create new problems such as overexertion or overdeveloped muscles. Bulging muscles may have suited man in the jungle, but they are not an asset to a desk worker. Furthermore, if this heavy brawn is to remain it must constantly be fed by vigorous body movements. Once you neglect these overdeveloped muscles, they sag and grow flabby.

No, brawn is not the answer for the modern man who must live a sedentary life. He needs the kind of movement that he can fit readily into a busy schedule. The requirements of the body for movement cannot be left only to week ends!

The modern man needs an antidote to his sedentary habits: sitting and turning in a swivel chair, leaning over a desk in a stoop-shouldered position, slumped back with feet on desk, slouched in an armchair viewing television. He has become accustomed to riding everywhere, to the train, up the stairs, to the shops. Thus, disused parts of the body become weakened. He eats well and drinks well, tending to become overweight. Is it any wonder that fatigue and backache result when the strain of this added weight is put upon muscles and joints weakened from poor use?

The Movement Schemes in this book provide the answer for the modern man. With them he can provide the body with movements which are a safe balance between too much and too little exercise. Even when done as exercises, the Movement Schemes take but little time, and make no demands in perspiration or fatigue. Furthermore, once the Movements are learned, they can be applied in normal activities: sitting, standing, bending, reaching. Thus they make no extra demands upon a busy day and they provide real relief from nervous tension.

If men realized the relationship between the shape of the body and the health of the body they would save themselves much grief. For a bulging abdomen and flabby waistline are signs of muscle weakness which may bring aches and pains, even serious bodily damage.

A physician of thirty-seven one day realized that something would have to be done about his backache. He found it almost too painful to stand at the operating table. (The medical diagnosis of his problem suggested that he might have a "prolapsed disc," a faulty alignment of the spine.) This physician was less aware of the flabby condition of his trunk, and how twisted his "middle area," the pelvis, was.

Our Movement Schemes aimed at strengthening the muscles guarding the back, and eliminating the strange twist in the "belt area." Within two months the pains were gone. Now the young physician, having seen his body day after day in the full mirrors at the Mensendieck Institute, became aware of his looks. We continued with most of the Movement Schemes in this book. One day he told us that his colleagues at the hospital had remarked: "You're looking quite the athlete these days!"

Thus functional movements answer special problems and the daily needs of modern man.

For Children

Parents will also find answers to many of the perplexing problems about guiding the development of the flexible bodies of their children:

> What is "good posture" and how is it achieved?
>
> Must there be the "awkward, clumsy phase" in growing children?
>
> What can be done to correct flat feet, weak ankles, bowlegs, knock-knees, crooked elbows, stooped shoulders, protruding shoulder blade wings?

What adjustments can be made in household furnishings to guard the shape of the young body?

With the Movement Schemes in this book, the parent can make the most of the impressionable characteristics of children. From the crib and the playpen they constantly observe and imitate adults, they learn how to move by copying adults.

From the porch of my house in Norway, I often used to watch with amusement a little boy about six years old. His father, who was the mayor, walked with his head down and his arms in back of him with hands clasped. The six-year-old always walked exactly the same way, arms clasped behind, head bent! One day I was surprised to find him walking with his head high. He continued to walk that way. Then I learned that his grandfather had come to visit. He was a fine old man renowned as a storyteller. He went from town to town telling folk tales. He replaced the father as the child's idol. And at the same time replaced the father as the child's model.

While I was the house guest of a young physician in Vienna, he asked me one day to go to his office to speak with him about something important. I couldn't imagine what it might be that he wanted to keep from his wife and adorable seven-year-old daughter. At the office he asked, "Did you notice anything about the child?"

19

I thought for a moment and said, "Are you referring to the child's lisp?"

"That's it!" he nodded. "What can I do about it?"

"Don't you know where it came from?" I asked somewhat amused.

He shook his head.

"It came from your wife."

"My wife?" he asked in astonishment.

"Weren't you aware of your wife's lisp?" I asked unbelieving.

"I am aware only of how lovely she is," he replied.

Unknown to us, the infant's eyes are like the sensitive feelers of radar. He registers most of the things we do. He may not understand them. He doesn't speak about them. But the image is implanted on his impressionable brain. How wonderful it would be, if during this impressionable age, all the adult movements he saw were natural, functional movements! What a difference it would make in building the foundation for a handsome figure, graceful movements and a healthy body!

From his earliest days, the child is forced to live in an adult world. Everything is too high for him: the chairs, the tables, the television set. He even has to look up at tall mother and tall father as he talks to them. If the child knew how to use his body correctly, he could compensate for the difficult physical environment. Nonetheless, something can be done to help him, in the home at least, by providing furnishings that enable him to sit in a restful position with back straight, shoulders squared, and head high. You will find some guideposts on suitable furniture in Chapter 3.

The Movement Schemes will reveal how futile some efforts are to encourage good posture in children without knowing how. What can a poor child do, for example, when her parent earnestly pleads, "Now sit up, Ann"? The chair is too high; the pillows are padded with springs! Ann might for the moment pull herself up, but the uncomfortable child would be straining and wasting her energy if she sat for long under such conditions.

Even assuming the chair is suitable, how helpful is it to say to a child, "Now sit up straight, don't hunch so! Push your shoulders back!" The child might snap into line stiffly, but she couldn't remain in that position long.

Furthermore, the instructions given to him in the hope of helping his body really do him little good. From the Movement Schemes comes the knowledge of how to help the child sit straight, stand straight, and in general use his body correctly.

If this help is given early, functional movements will become automatic and he will need little further guidance or reminders. IT IS AS EASY FOR THE CHILD TO LEARN TO USE HIS BODY CORRECTLY AS IT IS FOR HIM TO LEARN TO USE IT BADLY. The parent can be the wise counselor and the correct example.

Should there be any signs of muscular weakness as reflected in a crooked back, protruding shoulder blades, poorly shaped calves, the Movement Schemes can come to the rescue. At the Greenwich Academy for Girls in Connecticut, the children are photographed when first they arrive. They are given instruction weekly in the Mensendieck System to meet their special problems. New photographs are taken from time to time to show their progress.

Frequently, children with special problems come to the Mensendieck Institutes with their parents and go through the Movement Schemes together.

How easily and sensibly children take to the conscious use of muscles is illustrated by a five-year-old youngster. Being a mechanically-minded boy, he thought that everything moving had to have a motor to make it move; even the muscle actions during the Movement Schemes had to be audibly motorized.

He was fascinated to find his muscles in the mirror, interested to see his shoulder blades come closely together. He was very careful in placing his feet just so and to have his arms move absolutely straight forward or sideward. But every slightest motion was accompanied by the noise of a motor, starting, stopping, reversing or accelerating, according to the empo of his movements. This continued through a number of lessons, until we considered it time to intervene:

22

"Do you know, Eric, muscles do not have a motor which can be heard."

"What makes them move then?"

"Thinking. You think the movement, and that will make the muscles move."

A very serious and thoughtful little boy did the next Movement Scheme accurately and quite silently.

"It works! You are right, the motor is in my brain."

And no noisy reversing or accelerating was ever needed again.

Sometimes a child instinctively will seek support for weak muscles. A girl of ten, who had grown too fast, had of her own accord found a way of supporting her weak back. While doing her homework, she would sit on the floor in a corner of the room, using the converging walls to support her trunk. In this manner she replaced instinctively the lack of support from weakened long back muscles. After doing the appropriate Movement Schemes, she could again rely upon the adequate support of her long back muscles and serious trouble, possibly a crooked back, had been prevented.

Mensendieck Movement Schemes stress accuracy and consequently have—at first—to be done slowly. It is only natural that youngsters may find this boring and sometimes compromises have to be made with their natural impatience.

An eight-year-old boy attended the Mensendieck

Institute in order to improve his stoop-shouldered condition. He had failed in sports at school, and often complained about his feet. He was intelligent and was well aware of his weakness.

The difference in pace between the gymnastics he was used to and the slower execution of the Mensendieck Movement Schemes seemed to him rather tedious. We settled on a compromise. He could jump up and try to touch the ceiling frequently between the Movement Schemes. This not only introduced the element of fun but served to improve the weak muscles in question.

A few months later another test in sports was due at his school. When next he came to the Mensendieck Institute, we waited impatiently for a report. But he said nothing. Finally we could restrain our curiosity no longer.

"I passed with A's and B's."

"But why," we asked, "didn't you tell us?"

"I did not want to tell you," he replied. "I feared that you might get conceited."

For Older People

The Mensendieck Movement Schemes can be done by young and old alike. All can benefit from them. Movement Schemes provide answers to the bodily problems of older people, such as:

24

How can I provide the body with the movement it requires and at the same time avoid strain and fatigue?

Can some characteristics usually associated with advancing age be prevented or altered, namely the scrawny neckline, fatty bump on the nape of the neck, double chin?

Can I do anything about easy loss of breath and a sense of tiredness?

Can I avoid the sort of movements which overtake some, the unsteady walk, the wobbly knees, the shaky hand?

Of course, the sooner people bring the muscles of the body to full tonic condition, the better it is for their figure and health. But even if the body has been long neglected, the Movement Schemes can bring improvement.

Those in their seventies or eighties can do the Movement Schemes and benefit from them because they are natural movements. They do not strain the body. They can be done slowly, in fact should be done slowly. Furthermore, they can at first be done in the seated position. Thereafter, some can be done by holding onto a chair. Ultimately, they all can be done in the standing position.

That the Movement Schemes can be used with success, even in old age, was revealed by a woman of eighty-two. She could scarcely take a step. She complained about backache and could not even walk the few blocks from her home to the Mensendieck Institute. Accordingly, we progressed slowly, first doing the movements in the seated position and later in the standing position. Within a little while she could easily walk from her home to the Institute. One day when she arrived she was quite indignant. "Do you know what just happened to me?" she asked. "At the street crossing a man offered me his arm to help me across!"

For Convalescents

How moderate these movements are has been amply demonstrated by people convalescing from serious illnesses. Those with rheumatic hearts or other ailments usually come on the counsel of their physicians. One young man of twenty-eight recuperating from the serious effects of rheumatic fever, started the Movement Schemes while still confined to bed. We therefore first gave him the Movement Scheme for correct breathing which he could do in bed. Soon he was able to sit up. Gradually he recovered his full strength. Ultimately, he even played tennis! So enthusiastic did he become with the Mensendieck System that he became an instructor of the System in the Physical Education Department at Yale University.

Even more serious was the condition of a lawyer who was confined to an oxygen tent. His future life as well as his successful practice were at stake. Beginning again with breathing movements and progressing to others, he ultimately achieved complete recovery and joyfully took up golf again.

If these people could do the Mensendieck Movement Schemes, surely they are not too vigorous for anyone!

The Future of Your Body

You can take a hand in deciding the future of your body. We have charted the way for you in this book. No longer need you continue to allow vital muscles to deteriorate, thus failing to claim the graceful, healthy body that should be yours.

Get to know your body. You can do this best by looking at yourself candidly, without clothes, preferably between two full mirrors so that you can see both the front and the back. We have included in Chapter 2 a self-test with which you can check your body's characteristics. This will help show you what to look for, to judge your body and to identify improvements.

The Movement Schemes included in this book are adequate to meet most of the common bodily problems. They are presented in a special way which makes full use of the experience of many years at the

Mensendieck Institutes. Why not give about ten minutes a day to the Movement Schemes?

To what better, more important use can you put ten minutes of your day? It will bring added vitality because you will be using the body naturally, efficiently, and thereby conserving its energy. It will bring you a happier outlook, the sense of well-being that comes with knowing you look your best. You will have the peace of mind that comes with being in harmony with yourself and with your environment.

2.

THE SHAPE OF YOUR BODY

From their very first Mensendieck lesson, people begin to realize how little they know about their own body. In a sense, their body is almost a stranger to them. Standing, without clothes, between two full-sized mirrors, most of them see their full back view for the first time.

We immediately begin the Movement Schemes. From time to time, we point to the skeleton that has a prominent place in the room, and explain the movement in question with its help. Red strands of wool fastened from the hip to the thigh, for example, serve to explain the working of the muscle which contributes toward a firm and shapely thigh.

We take pains to explain such muscles because the shape of your body depends upon the condition of your muscles. Muscles, covering the framework of bone, give the body shape. The bones, like the beams of a house, provide the frame, but it is the muscle flesh that clothes the body. It is the "tonic" condition of the muscle that accounts for a slender contour at the hip, a rounded tight buttocks, a high firm breast, a tall erect line.

Therefore we must direct our attention to the muscles. Each muscle performs a function: one muscle group raises the arm, another expands the ribs, others hold the back erect, and some maintain the foot arch for sustaining the weight of the body. When each muscle performs the function nature intended and none other, when it is used adequately in this natural way, then the muscle is in good condition. We say the muscle is in "tonic" condition. Its elastic fibers contract easily, becoming shorter, thicker and harder. In this condition they readily provide the power we need. When we relax the muscle, if it is in tonic condition, its fibers readily return to their original position. The blood flows easily through such muscles and all parts of the body feel alive and strong.

But if the muscle is not used often enough, or not used properly, its condition deteriorates. The many fibers of the muscle like so many overstretched springs, contract less readily and remain loose. With disuse, layers of fat may form between them. Blood circulates poorly. All this is marked on the body and may be seen in a heavy ankle, a bulging abdomen, a flabby buttocks, puffy sides or a double chin.

Accordingly, the Movement Schemes aim at muscles—specific muscles in need of help. We aim to restore their tonic condition, thereby providing the attractive lines and vitality that the body should have.

That this can be done is one of the marvels of nature. For the natural healing powers of the body demonstrated when we cut a hand, break a bone or catch cold apply also to muscles. Even after years of abuse and neglect, muscles can be healed in the sense that they can be restored to natural tonic condition.

But to do this we must first identify the muscles in need of help, and aim our movements directly at them. If you cut your thumb, you wouldn't think of putting a bandage on your wrist. Similarly, if your thigh is heavy, you must reach the exact muscle group responsible. In the Mensendieck Institutes people are introduced to their bodies. By this means the muscles in need of help are identified. Their role in the body is clarified. And the movements to achieve their restoration carefully applied. Nature's restorative powers bear fruit thereafter.

In this chapter, we shall introduce you to your body as though you were at one of the Mensendieck Institutes. With the help of a self-test we have specially prepared, you will know better how to observe your body so that you can direct your aim accurately at the specific muscles in need of restoration. Finally, in this chapter, we will give several illustrations from actual experience to show how this knowledge of the body is applied in Movement Schemes.

Take Inventory of Your Body

Place two mirrors so that you get a full view of both the front and back of your body. If possible, use long mirrors. You can get the full back view by placing one mirror straight. Stand between it and the second mirror. Move the second mirror until you find the angle that enables you to see the whole back. (If you have only one mirror handy, make the most of it.)

Now step between the mirrors without clothes. Stand as you normally would in a "relaxed" position. The questions are aimed at getting information not only on the shape of your body, but also on how you use it.

The Feet and Legs

1. What is the position of your feet?
   a) Pointing toward each other at the toes.
   b) Pointing away from each other at the toes.
   c) Straight and parallel to each other.

2. On which part of the feet are you carrying the weight of the body?
   a) On the heels.
   b) Near the outer margin, below the little toes.
   c) Near the big toe, on the ball of each foot.

3. What is the condition of your ankles?

   a) Heavy.

   b) Slender.

   c) Crooked.

   What is the shape of your lower legs, that is the part between the ankles and knees?

   a) They bulge backward like a saber or crescent.

   b) They bend outward, bowlegs.

   c) The calves are heavy and thick.

   d) They taper evenly toward the ankle.

5. What is the condition of your knees?

   a) Knock-kneed.

   b) Straight.

   c) Pushed back.

   d) Heavy, thick, joint not visible.

6. Are your thighs

   a) Heavy?

   b) Firm and tapered?

   c) Flabby?

The Middle Area

7. When you bend the trunk forward, how do you manage the abdomen?

   a) It is relaxed and protrudes naturally.

   b) It is tight and flat.

   c) It is pushed out, rounded.

33

8. Are your buttocks
   a) Flabby, hanging?
   b) Tight and small?
   c) Heavy, highly rounded?

9. Is your abdomen
   a) Flat with a groove clearly visible down the middle through the navel?
   b) Heavy and bulging—the "bay window"?
   c) Slightly bulging, without middle groove?

10. Do you have
    a) Broad hips?
    b) Slender hips?

Shoulders and Upper Back

11. When you wish to straighten your shoulders, how do you do this?
    a) Push the shoulder tips backward.
    b) Pull the shoulder tips toward the ears.
    c) Draw the shoulders back by pulling with muscles in the middle of the back.

12. What is the condition of your back?
    a) Erect, upright, with muscle design visible.
    b) Stooped forward with "wings" protruding.
    c) Leaning backward, with ribs protruding in front.

13. Do your shoulders
    a) Droop sharply down at the sides—penguin shaped?
    b) Droop forward, narrowing the chest?
    c) Stand square, tapering slightly?

Neckline and Arms

14. When you bend and raise the head, which muscles of the neck do you use?
    a) The muscles in back of the neck.
    b) The muscles in front.
    c) The muscles at the sides.

15. Is your neck
    a) Evenly rounded and slender?
    b) Thick, bulgy, fatty?
    c) Thin and scrawny?
    d) At lower end in back, bumped by fat?

16. Is your head
    a) Straight?
    b) Leaning forward?
    c) Leaning sideways?
    d) Leaning back?

17. Concerning your neckline in general:
    a) It is hollow and scrawny near the collar bone.

b) The flesh hangs under the chin (double chin).

c) The Adam's apple protrudes.

d) It is filled in, smooth, the skin tightly drawn.

18. When you raise the arm forward and upward to shoulder height, where do your thoughts go to begin the lifting?

a) The shoulder tip.

b) The hand.

c) The elbow region.

19. With regard to the elbow, do you tend to hold it

a) Bent?

b) Straight?

c) Stretched so that the upper and lower arm form a slight v-shape?

20. Are your arms

a) Evenly rounded?

b) Flabby?

c) Thin?

d) Thick at the wrist joint?

These are the answers that would indicate you are using your muscles in accordance with functional movement, that therefore your body lines are graceful and attractive:

1c	6b	11c	16a
2c	7b	12a	17d
3b	8b	13c	18a
4d	9a	14a	19b
5b	10b	15a	20a

You will soon recognize why this is so from our discussion of the body and our application of the movement schemes.

Seven Basic Points About Muscles and Your Figure

1. *Muscles balance the body's parts.* One of the facts you will discover as you do the Mensendieck Movement Schemes is that you can, in a sense, juggle the parts of the body. You can line up the parts so that the body is tall and straight. Or you can let the parts tilt, so that the body leans forward, sideways or backward. You can let parts of the body fall out of line: the head may tilt to one side, one shoulder may hang lower than the other, a knee may bend dragging the hip down a bit.

In view of this, we have found it helpful to think of the body as being made up of principal parts fitting together by means of joints. Each part can be moved somewhat. Thus there are fourteen principal parts with differing weights as follows, assuming a person to weigh 150 pounds:

2	Feet	3 lbs. each	6 lbs.
2	Lower legs	7 lbs. each	14 lbs.
2	Thighs	15 lbs. each	30 lbs.
1	Trunk		70 lbs.
2	Upper arms	5 lbs. each	10 lbs.
2	Forearms	4 lbs. each	8 lbs.
2	Hands	1 lb. each	2 lbs.
1	Head	10 lbs.	10 lbs.
14			150 lbs.

While these fourteen parts are not separate in the sense that they can be moved around individually like the building blocks a child uses, they nonetheless can be moved singly within limits. These parts of the body are connected by joints, their smooth surfaces are held together by ligaments, tendons and muscles.

How wonderfully nature has adapted the size of the muscle to the job it has to do! The thigh muscle is large because it has to move about 25 pounds (for the person of 150 pounds). The shoulder-arm muscle is smaller, it has to move only 15 pounds.

These specially adapted muscles are in reality constantly balancing fourteen parts of the body throughout the day's activities. How you use the

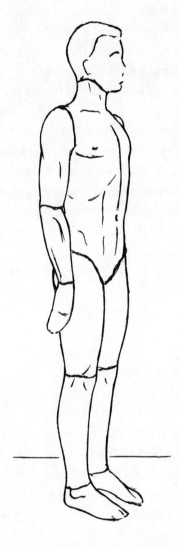

The weights of the body parts

muscles to do this job, therefore, helps determine the shape of the body.

2. *Muscles control the foot arch and create a strong foundation for the weight of the body.* The feet provide the foundation on which to balance the body in correct alignment. The condition of the feet and how they are used therefore becomes of great importance. Any weakness in the feet is easily transmitted to other parts of the body. So seemingly minor a thing as where you place the weight of the body upon the foot can determine whether the arch falls, the ankles thicken, the abdomen protrudes or the back aches.

The science of Body Mechanics indicates that the long arch extending from the heel to a point just before the big toe is best suited for carrying the weight of the body. But whether that arch is maintained depends upon the collaboration of several muscles.

This is why. The foot arch may be considered as being supported by two pillars. One pillar, the heel, is fixed and we need not worry about its doing its job. The second pillar we call the ball of the foot, the area around and including the big toe joint.

The ball of the foot is made to serve as a support for the weight by using the Peronaeus muscle. This muscle extends from the knee, along the outside of the lower leg, across the sole of the foot and is fastened near the ball of the foot. When being used, the Peronaeus muscle maintains the ball of the foot in place and thereby erects the second support for the arch. If this muscle is not used, the result may be falling arches or flat feet.

By carrying the weight of the body toward the ball of the foot while standing or walking, you bring the Peronaeus muscle into action. Distributing the weight of the body between the heel and the ball of the foot creates a reliable and elastic foundation for the body weight.

3. *Muscles hold the body upright.* The framework of bones and their joints would tumble to the ground if muscles did not draw them up into place and hold them there. To illustrate, when a large tree is transplanted, cords are fastened to pull in opposite directions to hold the tree erect until its roots take hold. The muscles pull similarly erecting the body upon a firm foot foundation. Some muscles pull from the front, others from the back, some from the right side, others from the left.

When the pull of these muscles is evenly balanced, the body stands erect. A muscle that is permitted to draw too hard moves a part out of line. But when the balance is achieved you see it in a tall, erect body. You feel it in the sense of harmony that pervades the body. The weight of the parts is evenly distributed. The right leg, for example, is carrying as much weight as the left. The buttock muscles assist the long back muscles in carrying the weight of the trunk.

If one part, however, is forced regularly to carry more than it should, unattractive body lines, even aches or pains may result. For example, if the long back muscles do not carry the weight of the trunk efficiently the result may be backache.

Therefore, each muscle must do its share in erecting the body, bringing to it harmonious lines and attractive balance.

4. *Muscles slenderize the body outline.* If the body is held erect on the firm foot foundation, many muscles contribute to slenderize the body outline. Nature has provided a goal toward which the muscles strive to draw the flesh. It is what we call the "Middle Line." This is a groove that runs down the center of the body. In front it passes down the abdomen through the navel. In back it runs down the center coinciding with the spine. This Middle Line divides the body into two equal halves.

The Middle Line is not always clearly visible. Only when the muscles are in tonic condition does the groove appear. Great sculptors have always recognized the Middle Line as an important indication of an attractively proportioned torso. You will often see a Middle Line on the sculptored masterpieces in museums.

If your own Middle Line is not now visible, it will gradually develop as you progress with the Movement Schemes. Its appearance will be a sign of the improvement in the shape of your body.

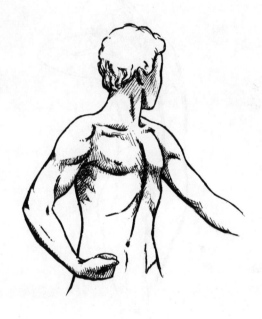

The Middle Line (Male)

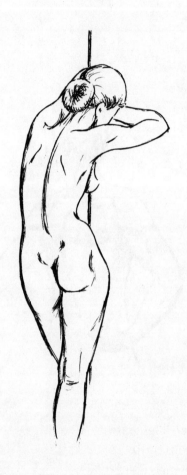

The Middle Line (Female)

The Middle Line marks the direction in which to draw the various body masses to render the body outline graceful and slender. There are muscles to do this along the thighs, the back and the neck. With these muscles each half of the body can be drawn toward the Middle Line. The result is a taller, more slender and graceful body outline.

5. *Muscles control the main center of gravity— the middle area.* Most people who become familiar with the Mensendieck Movement Schemes are surprised to discover that the buttocks are important for the shape of the body. Previously, they had tended to look upon this flesh as padding rather than muscle.

The appearance and health of the body are influenced by the buttock muscles. They help to strap the leg bones into the hip socket. Thus the buttocks influence leg movements such as walking, running and climbing. The condition of the buttock muscles determines the contours of the thighs at the hip, as well as the buttocks itself.

The strength of the lower back also depends upon the buttocks. This is the area where the long bony column, the spine, is joined with the wide bony belt, the pelvis. The buttocks hold this pelvis upright, thereby helping to avoid weak back, various general aches and such disturbances as sacroiliac or sciatica.

Furthermore, when the pelvis is held properly, it joins with the spine in guarding a straight back.

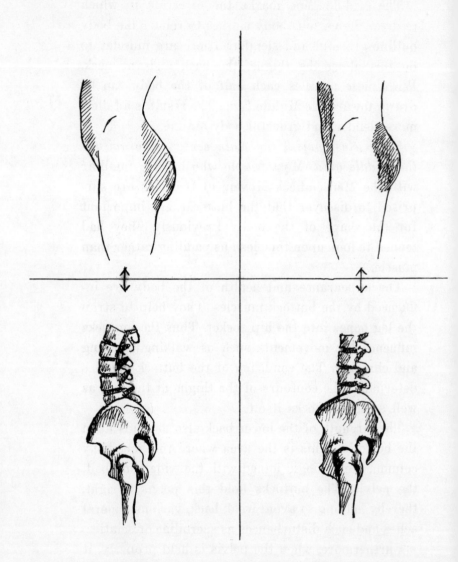

The muscles that shape the abdomen and buttocks

Meanwhile, other back muscles control the shoulders, squaring them with only a slight taper. They also hold the upper back flat. With this back foundation built upward by the buttocks, muscles at the upper back can help erect the head, thereby helping to avoid the unsightly "double chin." From this it can readily be seen that the buttocks govern the main center of gravity and are pivotal in shaping a graceful body, and assuring a healthy one.

6. *Muscles control the chest, its breathing apparatus and the breasts.* Few people realize that it is possible to improve breathing. Breathing enables fresh air and its oxygen to flow into the body, and waste air including toxic gases to escape from the body. Both inhalation and exhalation are accordingly of equal importance.

The apparatus nature has provided for this is truly remarkable. On the one hand the chest is a bony cage, strong and rigid enough to protect the vital organs, the heart and lungs. On the other hand, it is a flexible cage, for muscles can move the bony ridges, permitting the lungs to expand and to contract.

The greater the expansion of this bony cage— the thorax—the more oxygen is taken in. By developing the muscles that interlace the bones of the cage we can increase our breathing capacities, and thereby eliminate easy loss of breath.

There is another benefit from proper use of these

muscles of the thorax. They can shape the upper chest, holding it high and bringing an added handsome line to the body.

Other muscles are also important for the chest. One runs from the upper arm along the collar bone over the chest. When in tonic condition this muscle smooths part of the neckline near the collar bone, preventing scrawniness there. It molds the chest. It supports the weight of the breasts, holding them higher.

7. *Muscles flatten the abdomen and hold the abdominal organs in place.* Many who come to the Mensendieck Institute are disturbed by the bulge of their abdomen. Yet few realize that this is basically a problem of muscle development.

Nature has equipped the body with a long abdominal muscle. It runs from the groin to the chest. This muscle serves as a wall. It holds the abdominal organs such as the digestive tract and the reproductive organs in place. The weight against this wall is heaviest at the lower end. If the muscle becomes weak from inadequate use, it can no longer hold the contents of the abdomen in place. The result, a bulging abdomen. This also affects the functioning of the abdominal organs.

By adequate movement, the abdominal muscles can be developed to perform the function of an abdominal wall. The result is a flat and youthful frontal outline.

The Seven Basic Points Applied

After childbirth, the abdominal muscles sag. A young mother of two children came one day to the Mensendieck Institute in a very unhappy state. Seventeen months earlier she had delivered her second child, and since then her body seemed to deteriorate. This didn't happen to other women having several children, she complained. It hadn't happened to her after the first child. Why should she now have to wear dresses sizes larger, and at the age of thirty-two have to use a corset?

We, too, were surprised that the deterioration had taken place so early. Usually, if one doesn't use natural, functional movements it becomes noticeable in the early forties. But the signs were unmistakably clear in the contours of her trunk: flabby folds down the sides and around the lower back; a protruding abdomen. There were many other signs: in the ankles, breasts, back of the neck. They all added up to this: the woman had not been very active in her youth, and such movement as she did give the parts of the body was haphazard.

We undertook to repair this with the Movement Schemes presented in this book. We aimed first to restore nature's wonderful "corset" of muscles which easily can hold the abdomen flat, the long muscle running from the groin to the chest with other layers of elastic muscle meeting it from the sides.

A study of anatomy and body movement had long convinced me that a way could be found to reach each of these abdominal muscles. Only by functional movements would they remain strong yet flexible, and thereby hold the abdomen flat. Two basic Movement Schemes presented in this book were the answer. One is the Abdominal Control movement. The other is the Side Stretch.

These were the very movements that worked so well for this young mother. She did them slowly and carefully between mirrors. In about a month there were signs of the tightening and shaping of the abdominal muscles.

One day she observed, and quite rightly, that the movements of the Side Stretch were entirely new to her. (How many of us have occasion to bend the trunk sideways? For this reason, it is desirable to do the Side Stretch at least twice during the day.)

She also observed that other Movement Schemes could be readily applied in her daily activities. Thus the full benefit of the Abdominal Control Movement Scheme could be obtained if its steps were followed whenever bending of the trunk was required.

The young mother did the other Movement Schemes for the waistline given in this book. Her delight in seeing the gradual change taking place in her body outline was justified. Within another month a substantial change had taken place. Progress continued until she had sculptured a truly graceful body.

Heavy thighs, the problems of a dancer. An attractive woman of twenty-nine was in great distress. She was attractive—that is, until you looked at her thighs. These were her undoing. So self-conscious of them had she become that she had given up her job as instructor of ballroom dancing. She withdrew into herself, eliminating most of her social life.

How great an impact one's looks can have upon the whole personality! The mirror tells no lies. It can smother us with a sense of inferiority, engulf us in a sea of depression. The constant feeling that we should do something to help ourselves keeps us in an unhappy mental state. This is probably the explanation of the "dividend" most people report when they do the Movement Schemes. For they are taking effective steps to improve their body's faults. They find themselves happier, more at peace with themsleves.

This dancer suffered not only from disfigurement, but from serious depression also. She felt "fate" had been unfair. This was understandable, for oddly enough she had given her legs considerable attention in her youth. She had been an avid student of ballet for several years. This involved rigorous training for the difficult ballet movements.

With the help of a skeleton for demonstration purposes, and strands of red wool to imitate the function of muscles, she soon realized that responsibility rested with herself and not "fate." Thigh muscles were heavier than other muscles of the body because

51

they had the difficult job of moving the legs while about seventy pounds of trunk weight rested on them. But she had developed exceptionally strong thigh muscles in her ballet dancing. Then, one day, she gave up ballet. She turned to the less strenuous movements of ballroom dancing. The strong thigh muscles scarcely were used.

What happened to this dancer happens to many people, but the results for her were exaggerated. The sag of flesh on the body, whether of the thighs or abdomen, is a sign that muscles which depend upon movement for their health are being left idle. In her case the muscles had been overdeveloped, so they sagged all the more.

But she felt that she had not neglected the thigh muscles since a year earlier when she first noticed their flabby condition. She had gone to a gymnasium. Then she had used massage. She had even returned to strenuous dance instruction, doing dance movements about two hours a day!

This dancer didn't realize two things. The damage had been done, specific muscles had been neglected. Secondly, movement alone was not enough. It had to be functional movement. It had to reach specific, weakened muscles.

Anatomy and the science of body mechanics pointed the way. The Movement Scheme I call the Leg Pendulum, Sideways had resulted and proved that movements could be devised to reach the specific muscles which now were the source of this dancer's troubles.

By the tenth day almost an inch had been taken off each thigh. Here, again, was a movement that did not occur frequently in one's daily activities. Do you move your leg sideways normally? Our dancer set aside five minutes each day to do this Movement Scheme three times with each leg. Within a few months their natural lines had been restored.

Aged sixty-three, and the pains came. This is an unusual case but it illustrates an important point. A man of sixty-three who was a government executive came to the Mensendieck Institute. The look in his eyes was one of resignation to a sad future, the lines around his mouth those of pain. His steps were short.

His story is in part the story of so many these days. Science has made our lives easy and wonderful, but we have failed to take the precautions to assure the enjoyment of its wonders in good health. We move on the wheels of an automobile, we spend long hours in the comforts of rubber foam pillows before television sets. Rather than work the fields or the mines, our chores are light and are frequently done by machines. Many of us spend eight hours a day hunched over a desk. Yet we take no special measures to give the body the movement it needs for good health, and we ignore the signs provided by flabby contours.

One morning the man reached to tie his shoelace and it was as though a thousand bolts of pain had been fired at his back and down his legs. Diathermy, health baths, potions—these and other cures were tried, until one orthopedic surgeon suggested correct bodily movement.

Since the man was sixty-three and in pain, it was necessary to proceed slowly. But one advantage of these natural Movement Schemes is that they conform wholly to the functioning of the body and accordingly are so mild that people of all ages can do them. He did them first in the seated position or holding on to the back of a chair. Within a month he could report taking steps without pain. Progress continued.

Our executive couldn't understand why this had happened to him. He had always been careful, and didn't remember suffering any injuries. Then we pointed to the skeleton which reveals so much about our bodies. He wanted the full story so that he could understand what had happened, what he would have to do and why.

I pointed to the long bony column in the center of the back. He was surprised that the little round sections of bone called vertebrae that made up the spinal column actually were separate. They were held together by muscle and other tissue. This made the spine flexible, the muscle doing the job of moving the spine.

Moving down to the lowest part of the spine, we came to the center for most of our executive's difficulties. The haven for many aches: sacroiliac, slipped discs, sciatica. The last five sectors of the spine are called the lumbar vertebrae. Below the lumbar vertebrae is a bone shaped like a shield. It is called the sacrum. This shield is part of nature's bony corset known as the pelvis. The other parts in the pelvis corset are the hip bones.

Our executive became a bit impatient with these explanations. No one likes to be spoken to in a language that is new, whether it be the language of Tibet or of Science. So we dropped the technical terms and went to the source of the backache.

Strands of muscle have the job of keeping all these separate bones tightly in place. At the same time muscles move the bones whenever body movement is required. The key then to a healthy back is to keep these muscles in tonic condition. If we don't, the several separate bones in the lower back may rub, though ever so slightly, as the pressure from the trunk of the body weighs heavily upon them. This may bring pain, as it did to our official. But this is a part of the body that few people move correctly in daily activities. That is why those Movement Schemes aimed at this critical area are so important. For many of the pains that originate here are transmitted up the back and down the legs.

The Movement Schemes which were particularly

55

helpful to our executive were the Back Stretch and the Leg Pendulum, Forward, Backward and Sideways. At the end of about seven months he walked normally and without pain.

3.

GUARDING THE BODY AT WORK, AT PLAY AND AT REST

Each movement of a day's activities is recorded on the body. The manner in which the various parts of the body are used, good or bad, leaves its imprint on the body structure and on its outline.

Perhaps, during the day, your shoulders were pushed too far upward while ironing on too high a board, or your back stooped too far forward while washing in a basin placed too low. During a period of relaxation in an easy chair, your lower back was perhaps curved in excess, the chest held hollow or the neck and head bent too far forward. All of these wrong movements and postures are registered on the body.

Any continued occupational posture when wrongly executed will bring its own harmful results. The dentist bends at his work all day, mostly to one side. Thus the weight of his body presses heavily on one leg, the back is twisted, and the head inclined unnaturally forward.

The child may be told to do his homework on the

high dining room table. His feet dangle from the large chair, while his back and shoulders strain to adjust themselves to furniture built to adult dimensions. He squirms to find a comfortable position, and finally puts his elbow on the table, resting his head in the palm of his hand, napping. The mother, pained at the sight of his rounded shoulders and protruding shoulder blade wings, is at a loss for an explanation of them. How could she know the home furniture is exacting such a high toll on her child's health?

The busy executive sits on a padded swivel chair which he can rock into several "comfortable" positions. The reports and letters which flow across his desk absorb all his attention. Perhaps he gives no thought to his posture. His lower back is hunched over, the abdomen protrudes, the trunk weight rests incorrectly on the pelvic bones. Then one day the unsightly contours of his abdomen distress him, or even worse, sacroiliac or sciatic conditions pain him. How could he know that the height of his desk and improper use of the swivel chair play havoc with his back and neck?

The housewife, having used her body wrongly in many of her housekeeping duties, is surprised at the hunched outline of her shoulders, the hollow back, the thickening legs. How could she know to relate these conditions to the height of the work surfaces in the kitchen? Yet she spends several hours a day preparing meals. During this time the body is registering the movements of the back, the neck and the head as she adjusts these to the height of the work surface when she mixes a batter or peels potatoes.

The answer for all such people, for anyone seeking graceful lines, health and vitality throughout the years is: KNOW YOUR BODY, and KNOW HOW TO USE IT WISELY. The basic facts are simple. We have already examined some of them.

In this chapter let us look more precisely at what we can do to guard the body throughout the day. The Movement Schemes will apply functional movements to your daily activities to assure that you bend, reach, walk and run in ways that will sustain or improve your body's looks and health. In addition to such movements, however, much of our day usually is spent in milder activity from the seated and standing positions.

In this chapter we shall determine how the body should best be used when we are seated and standing. We shall arrive at some rules for achieving the Balanced Seated Position, and the Balanced Standing Position. Aside from their application throughout the day, these will be important to you when you turn to do the Movement Schemes.

How we stand or sit during the day can be influenced greatly by our home, office and shop furnishings. Therefore, in this chapter, we also shall discuss chairs, desks and work surfaces to assure that these assist you in guarding the body. We shall notice how these furnishings and the way you use them can determine whether you achieve adequate bodily rest and relaxation, and accordingly release from fatigue and nervous tension. The role played by diet, exercise and athletics in shaping the body is also examined.

How to Sit in Balance

Ordinarily, we sit in a chair to rest the body while at work, while we dine and when we relax the mind— by reading, for example. Whether the body actually is being rested depends upon the way we sit, the way we use the chair. Furthermore, the way we sit affects the shape and health of the body.

The structure of the body points the way to the correct sitting position. The human anatomy reveals that we have been provided with "sitting bones." These are the curved ridges of bone at each side of the lower edge of the bony belt called the pelvis. The two curved ridges of bone can be likened to the curved rockers of a rocking chair. The trunk may rock on the sitting bones, or it may be stopped and held still on its balancing point as would a rocking chair.

Find your sitting bone in this way.

Sit toward the front edge of a chair without

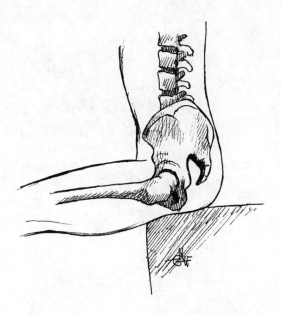

The sitting bones and the health of the back

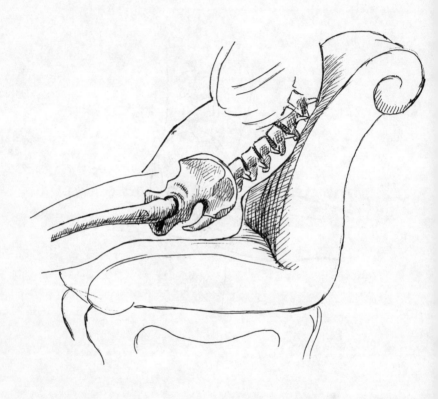

How you sit affects the shape of the body and the health
of the back

arms or padding, such as the ordinary kitchen chair.

Let your feet rest flat on the ground.

Hold your back straight.

Slide your left hand, palm upward, under your buttocks on the left side; that is, between the buttocks and the chair. Place your right hand similarly.

Move the fingers until you feel a bony ridge pressing against the fingers. This bony ridge is the sitting bone.

Now rock the trunk forward and backward on the sitting bone. Sense how the pressure on the fingers increases and decreases depending upon the position of your trunk. When the pressure on the fingers is greatest you are using the proper point on the sitting bones for balancing the trunk. It is comparable to the exact spot on the rocking chair which will balance it and thus hold it steady.

The reason this exact point on the sitting bone is so important is that the position of the back, shoulders, chest and abdomen depend upon it. With the weight of the body directed to this point, the pelvis is held erect and the trunk weight above it may be maintained in the correct, balanced position. This is the basis for the Balanced Sitting Position.

Nine Steps in Assuming the Balanced Sitting Position

1. *Sit toward the front edge of the chair.* Only by sitting toward the front of the chair can you assure proper use of the sitting bones. Otherwise you will be sitting partly on your thighs, drawing the back out of line.

2. *Place both feet flat and parallel on the ground, a few inches apart.* The feet serve as a good foundation for the body even in the sitting position. Have the feet flat on the floor, straight and parallel to each other and about three inches apart. The pressure should be directed at the area back of the big toe including the big toe joint. This, you remember, is the ball of the foot.

3. *Use the sitting bones.* With some practice, you can readily know when you are seated on the balancing point of the sitting bones. It will be the spot where the pressure of the sitting bone is greatest against the chair.

4. *Hold the knees parallel.* With the legs bent, have the knees face straight forward and about three inches apart.

5. *Press lightly onto the ball of each foot, and onto the sitting bones.*

6. *Draw the head and trunk up tall and straight.* With the long back muscles, slowly stretch the spine straight upward toward the center of the head, the "crown" of the head.

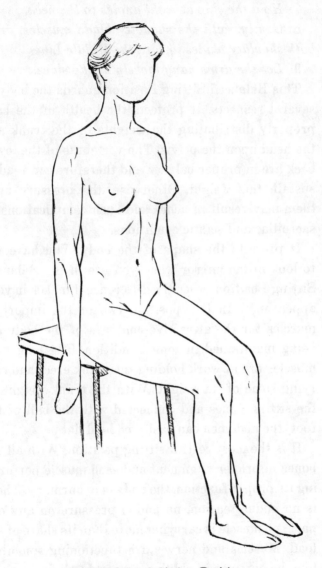

The Balanced Sitting Position

7. *Hold the chin at right angles to the neck.*

8. *Gently, with the shoulder blade muscles, draw both shoulder blades toward the Middle Line.*

9. *Let the arms hang loosely at the sides.*

This Balanced Sitting Position guards the body in several respects. It protects the health of the back properly distributing the weights of the trunk and the head upon the pelvis. The vertebrae of the lower back are in proper balance and therefore can readily sustain this weight. Otherwise, the pressure upon them may result in aches and such complications as sacroiliac and sciatic conditions.

It protects the shape of the body. You have but to look in the mirror when you are in the Balanced Sitting Position to see the difference it makes in your appearance. In this position two of the important muscles for the attractive contours of the body are being maintained in tonic condition. The long back muscles are at work holding the trunk erect and carrying some of its weight. With the trunk weight on the sitting bones and connected with the ball of the foot, the abdomen can easily be held flat.

It is the most restful sitting position. With all the bones in proper alignment and each muscle performing its proper function, the body is in harmony. There is no undue tension, no undue pressure on any one part; no muscle is carrying more than its share of the load. Muscles and nerves are functioning smoothly, like the oarsmen in rhythm, smoothly gliding a shell.

It is conducive to good breathing, a straight spine and eliminates all harmful pressures on the lumbar region and the back of the thighs. It prevents sacroiliac or sciatic pains. Under normal muscular conditions, the Balanced Sitting Position can be assumed easily, almost without conscious effort. It is not strenuous to hold the trunk erect in this posture. Once fully accustomed to it, you will find the balanced position more relaxing than any deviation from it.

While at first it may require attention to sit this way, gradually sitting in balance will become automatic. The pillowed easy chair, the source of so much damage to your body, may even lose its attraction for you.

How to Stand in Balance

It is wise also to know how to conserve energy and avoid fatigue while standing. This is particularly so for those who have to work in the standing position most of the day. Standing in balance facilitates economy of movement, thereby reducing fatigue and the frictions that produce aches and pains in joints and muscles. It activates those muscles which should be at work holding the body erect, thereby helping to keep them in tonic condition.

The science of body mechanics points the way also to the Balanced Standing Position. Standing in balance calls for the proper distribution of the weights of the body through the correct alignment of the body parts. The muscles must be so controlled as to assure this alignment.

The body weight should be directed toward the front of the foot, along its inner margin, so that it is carried not only by the heel but also by the ball of the foot. Only by directing the weight toward the ball of the foot can you maintain the long foot arch. This arch sustains the weight of the body without weakening the foot. You can assure the use of the ball of the foot by having the feet straight and parallel to each other, a few inches apart. On this correct foundation the legs and trunk can readily be held in proper alignment.

To hold the legs and trunk straight, two joints have to be controlled: the ankle joint and the knee joint. This is done by maintaining an equal muscle action in front and in back of the legs. You will thereby control the leg bones at the two joints, holding the legs straight.

The buttock muscles are important for the proper alignment of the trunk on the legs since the buttocks control the hip joint. They help maintain the pelvis in balance within the hip joint and thereby provide the base for a straight back. Movement Scheme 3 will show you how to control the buttocks.

You stretch the trunk up tall and straight by means of the long back muscles on either side of the spine. This will give you the sensation that you are

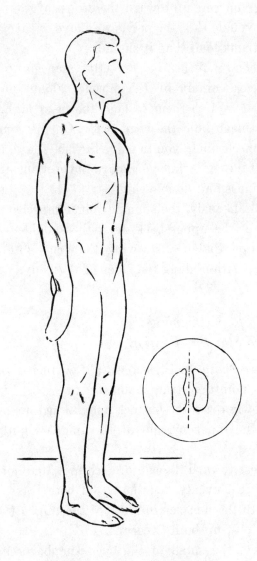

The Balanced Standing Position

pulling yourself up toward the crown of your head. Unless you do this, the pelvis will have to carry more of the trunk load than it should.

The head will then be correctly balanced upon the erect neck column by the muscles along the back of the neck. Use them to hold the head high. This doesn't mean hold the head stiffly. On the contrary, these muscles help you to move the head more gracefully. At the same time you guard the neckline against scrawniness and double chin.

Simultaneously, the shoulder blade muscles at the middle of the upper back draw the shoulder girdle into proper balance, drawing the arms into their correct position along the sides of the body.

Eight Steps in Assuming the Balanced Standing Position

1. Place both feet parallel, a few inches apart, big toes pointing straight ahead.

2. Slowly draw the buttock and Adductor muscles (along the inner margin of the thigh) tightly together.

3. Press toward the ball of each foot, and hold the body weight evenly distributed on both legs.

4. With the muscles in front of the thighs (Quadriceps), pull up both kneecaps.

5. From the small of the back (lumbar region), with the long back muscles, slowly stretch the back

straight upward. Draw yourself up toward the "crown" of the head.

6. Simultaneously, gently move the chin slightly forward until it is held at right angles to the front of the neck.

7. From the center of the upper back, with the shoulder blade muscles (Rhomboideus and Trapezius), slowly draw the shoulder blades back and down until they are flat and held together.

8. Let the arms hang loosely at the sides.

This standing position should be used to guard the body throughout the day. You can use it when you stand waiting for a train, bus, elevator, or while talking with another person. It is the most restful standing position for the body is not held rigid, yet is in perfect balance with all muscles functioning properly.

You can use it also when you have to stand at some chore or at your work. The girl behind the counter, the workman at his bench, the artist at his easel, the policeman, the orchestra conductor—all will derive special benefit from standing in balance.

There is a useful variation on the Balanced Standing Position to enable ready movement. Place the feet in step position; that is, one foot forward as though you were about to take a step. With the feet in this position you can reach and move more readily, shifting the weight easily from one foot to the other.

The ease with which you stand in balance and sit in balance depends upon the condition of your muscles. As you do the Movement Schemes in this book you will improve the long back muscles, the buttocks, the shoulder-blade muscles—all of which play so important a part in the way you stand and sit. In this way you will really sit and stand in comfort for you will be using all of your muscles properly, thereby resting the body—reducing unnecessary nerve and muscle action. You will also be comfortable in the knowledge that as you sit and stand you are guarding the shape of the body also.

Furniture to Guard Your Body's Health and Looks

Whether we can readily assume the Balanced Sitting Position and the Balanced Standing Position frequently depends upon the furnishings of the home, the office, the workshop. The height of a chair, work surface or desk should be such that the body does not have to make adjustments harmful to its structure and outline.

The restful chair. The Balanced Sitting Position establishes these characteristics for the truly restful chair. Its height enables your feet to remain flat on the floor and your thighs parallel to the floor when you sit toward the front edge of the chair. Since the length of the legs of members of the family vary, the height of the chairs in the household should also vary.

The upholstery of a truly restful chair should be neither too soft nor too hard. It should enable you readily to find the proper point on the sitting bone. The buttock muscles provide adequate padding to assure comfort. If some chair padding is required, it should be without springs. They are an uncertain foundation on which to hold the trunk erect.

The healthful chair need not have arms, for in the Balanced Sitting Position additional support for back or arms is unnecessary. It is difficult to find arm rests at a suitable height, one that enables you to keep the shoulders back and low. To preserve a normal, attractive shoulder outline and to relax the arm muscles, allow the hands to rest in the lap.

When your long back muscles are sufficiently strong to hold the trunk erect, the chair back becomes unnecessary—except for weak or elderly people. When you lean against the back of a chair, your weight is incorrectly distributed. The position of the pelvis is disturbed and the lower back is curved outward too far. This prevents the muscles from holding the abdomen flat.

Complete relaxation for all parts of the body cannot be obtained in the seated position. In order to relax completely, it is best to lie down, on a couch, on the floor or on a bed, whenever the opportunity pre-

73

sents itself. To achieve complete rest, the body has to be supported in all its parts. The couch or bed should be firm enough to offer sufficient "rebound." Springs may be too elastic to provide the right support.

The table. Having decided upon the characteristics of a suitable chair, we now can relate them to the table. Here the important factor is to be sure that the height of the table enables you to keep the shoulders back and down. This is particularly so for writing tables. You can determine when a table is the proper height for your body in this way. Sit in a chair in the Balanced Sitting Position close to the table. Bend your elbow. With the shoulders back and down, the bent elbow should just touch the table top. When the table is this height, you can rest the forearm upon it assured that you are guarding your shoulder line.

Adapting your body to an unsuitable table will spoil the shoulder and neck lines. If carried on over a long period of time, it will result in fatigue and tension along the neck and upper back.

The relationship of the chair to the dining table invariably causes problems for children. The seat is too low. Accordingly, the child is propped up on pillows or books. The child's feet dangle, making it difficult to use the sitting bone properly. One solution is to have a special child's chair. This is high enough so that his bent elbow can rest on the table top. A hinged platform attached to the legs of the chair at the proper height enables the child to place his feet flat upon it, thus providing the required foot support for the Balanced Sitting Position.

Kitchen and other home furnishings. Since the woman spends so much time in the kitchen, the furnishings and equipment found there become very important in terms of avoiding fatigue and preserving an attractive, healthy figure. Of primary importance in the kitchen is the height of the work surfaces, particularly those on which she prepares the food and irons the clothes. The proportions of her body provide the key to the correct height of these surfaces. You can determine the height in this way. Stand in the Balanced Standing Position, the step forward variation, close to the work surface. The top of this surface should reach the wrist. At this level, the shoulders will remain back and low as the various kitchen jobs are being done, whether cleaning vegetables or ironing clothes. In order to be able to stand in the step position, that is with one foot forward, the area under the work surface should be free. This will enable you to stand in balance closer to the table, and to reach or turn with greater ease.

Perhaps the kitchen in your house or apartment does not wholly meet these requirements. Nonetheless, it is desirable that you have a work surface that meets your needs, even if it provides only a two-foot-square area. A chopping board this size fastened with flanges to four pieces of pipe the proper length provides a practical and inexpensive kitchen work surface. In any case, it's well worth the small expense involved to save the nerves and figure of the housewife.

Kitchen furnishings should also include a suitable stool to enable the woman to sit at her work whenever possible. The height of the stool is such that the woman when in the seated position can have her elbow touch the surface while holding the shoulders back and down. A platform fastened to the stool legs at proper height enables the feet to be held forward in the Balanced Sitting Position. Incidentally, the seat of the stool should be square with rounded edges, rather than circular, since the square seat provides a better surface for the sitting bone and thigh.

The beds in the home are important for proper rest. A proper mattress and spring combination facilitates rest. A firm bed enables you to relax your muscles throughout the body, for it is being supported on an even level. Otherwise, a hip, a shoulder or the lower back may sink into the mattress bringing muscles into action to support the body level. An even mattress is important for these reasons.

A reading stand would be a valuable addition to any household. This enables you not only to guard the eyes, but the neckline, the shoulder line and many muscles of the upper back. A stand similar to a musician's stand could be used. Its height adjusted, its distance from the eyes adjusted, you could then sit straight and keep the correct posture of the head, shoulders and upper back. It would prevent fatigue and continued eyestrain.

Finally, the home should make greater use of mirrors, particularly in the kitchen and the living room. These would help remind you to guard the body by using the Balanced Sitting Position and the Balanced Standing Position.

One final observation about home furnishings. The body is sufficiently supple so that everything m the house need not be at easy arm's reach. Each time you bend or reach to get things, you actually are giving the body an opportunity to perform a functional movement. This means you can have drawers and bookshelves near the floor, and storage space near the ceiling in closets. If you use this storage space often enough it should be at a height you can reach by stretching.

Furnishings of the office, shop, etc. Each occupation involves hazards for the body, unless special precautions are taken in the use of the body and in the furnishings which affect the use of the body. The desk of the executive and the chair of the typist may be hazards. The position of the music stand and the demands of the cello upon the arm may be hazards. The desks in the schoolroom, the switchboards of telephone operators, the change counters in banks, the work tables in shops, all of these may be hazards.

The Balanced Sitting Position and the Balanced Standing Position provide us with yardsticks for determining how to minimize or eliminate these hazards.

The height and arrangement of office furniture is important because men and women sit at desks for long periods of time. To mention just one case in point, a woman in her mid-twenties began to feel severe pains in her back. Her back was crooked, and one shoulder slanted down. She was a secretary whose working arrangement was such that, while seated before a typewriter, she constantly had to reach for materials in a set of shelves on her right. She also had to lean over and reach for files in a cabinet near the floor.

Rather than facilitate these movements the office furnishings hindered them. The typewriting table was such that she couldn't get her feet under it. She didn't have a swivel chair, so she constantly twisted her body. Along with the Movement Schemes to help remedy her condition, we emphasized the importance of the Balanced Sitting Position. She readily recognized the need for having the office furnishings changed so that she could maintain this position. A small swivel chair enabled her thereafter to rotate without twisting her body. A little back rest at the lower back helped relieve the long back muscles during the period they were being strengthened. Another typewriting table enabled her to sit in the balanced position, having the correct height and space underneath for her feet.

The furniture used by the executive must meet his special needs. The swivel chair which has so many attractive features for the busy executive can be harmful if its seat is too high off the ground. If the leather upholstery causes the edge of the seat to taper, the sitting bones can not be properly used. This will cause the lower back to bulge, resulting in fatigue and backache.

The height of the desk affects the shape of the shoulders and the condition of the upper back and neck. The proper height permits his elbows when bent to touch the desk top. This makes it possible for him to write without shoving his shoulders up and out of line. A reading stand also helps him reduce fatigue and at the same time guard the neckline.

Factory work usually makes strong physical demands on the body. Therefore it is all the more important that the working conditions help conserve the energy and guard the bodies of workers. Workers are showing increasing concern with these matters. At one of the Mensendieck Institutes in Sweden, workers gather once a week to perform the Movement Schemes in order to learn how to use their bodies wisely, protecting their health and vitality.

The Balanced Sitting Position and the Balanced Standing Position are important in the factory. If the worker is seated at a machine all day, the height of the machine and seat should be brought into proper relationship. This enables him to maintain the Balanced Sitting Position. With the height of the machine such that his bent elbow touches the top surface, his shoulders can be held properly.

If the worker stands all day and adjustments can not be made in the height of the work surface to enable him to stand in balance, then a platform can be supplied. This would enable him to stand at his work so that his wrist is even with the top of the work table. There should be ample leg room under the table to enable him to stand in the step position.

Whenever possible, people should sit at their work, or at least sit at intervals during the day. Salespeople in department stores, elevator operators and factory workers can be provided with stools enabling them to sit at their work, or when they have the chance. The height of the stool should be related to the work surface so that the bent elbow can rest on the top. If the feet cannot remain flat on the ground, the stool should have a platform.

Nervous Tension and Fatigue, Rest and Relaxation

Whether at home or at work, we all at some point in the daily cycle of activities seek rest and sleep. However, the use we make of the body greatly influences the rate at which we become tired and fatigued. It also affects the condition of the nervous system and whether we become nervously tense during the day.

We can understand what is happening if we look upon the body as a marvelously equipped communication system. Every part of the body is "wired" by nerves. These nerves stretching throughout the body are connected with the main trunk line of nerves, the spinal column. All nerves are linked to the highly sensitive area, the brain.

The brain is constantly receiving messages over the nerves and dispatching messages. When the thought is formed in the brain, "Reach for the book," messages in properly synchronized order are sent to the muscles via the nerves. "Shoulder arm muscles raise the arm. Upper arm muscles bend the arm at the elbow. Forearm muscles move the fingers." And the book is grasped. All this happens in a split second. Thus the nerve system and muscle system are intimately linked.

In a telephone system, each home has its wire and number. When you dial an exact number, say 7171, the phone rings at your friend's home. If meanwhile, someone else rings 7171, he gets a busy signal.

Similarly, in the body each muscle has a function. It is hooked up with nerves via which instructions for the action are received. To lift the arm requires the sending of messages over specific nerve "wires" to specific muscles.

If you wish to raise your arm and your thoughts

flow to the hand and the shoulder rather than the shoulder alone, the channels of your nervous system become unnecessarily clogged. Additional nerves are transmitting messages. Additional muscles are being used. When the message, "Reach for the book," goes to the hand, there are "busy signals." Multiply this by hundreds of times to take into account all the messages being received and dispatched via the nerves, and you can see the strain on the nervous system which incorrect body movement causes. There are constant "busy signals," "repeated wrong numbers," "continuous buzzings."

This comparison with the telephone system cannot be carried too far. The idea is simply this. Each muscle has a function. Specific nerves serve each muscle. If the correct muscle is being used for the intended movement then the message from the brain flows smoothly. If more muscles are being used than necessary for a movement, it means more nerves are being used. If wrong muscles are being used, it means muscles and nerves stand by ready to do the job but are not being used.

Proper nerve use and nerve control are closely linked with muscle use and muscle control. Harmonious use of muscle results in harmony within the nervous system, and consequently a reduction in nervous tension.

The Movement Schemes in this book are aimed at achieving muscle control. It is clear from the anatomy of the body that muscle control is linked with nerve control. Thus the Movement Schemes will bring nerve control and accordingly an easing of nerve tension. Throughout the day, as you perform movements functionally, you will sense this reduction in nervous tension.

Aside from its effect on the nerves, muscle control reduces fatigue. While in the course of the day's activities muscles become tired and the body fatigued, there are ways to reduce fatigue and thereby increase your vitality. The body can sustain itself through the day's work without the sense of crushing fatigue some people feel. Proper rest and relaxation can also help overcome fatigue.

Correct use of muscles requires not only that the right muscle be used for a specific action, but also that the muscle be "relaxed" from time to time. The skilled oarsmen in a team set up a rhythm that goes "Stroke—glide, stroke—glide." If the rhythm went "Stroke, stroke, stroke, stroke," the bodies of the oarsmen could not take the strain.

So many of us "stroke, stroke, stroke" in our use of muscles when we could so readily "stroke—glide—stroke." This would overcome fatigue. It would also increase our efficiency.

This is particularly important when we realize that we can only rest the entire body when we lie down. Yet how many of us can lie down in the course of a busy day? Therefore, we must find the means of resting the body without lying down. Even so mild an activity as sitting keeps some muscles on the job. Nonetheless, there are ways to give many muscles a rest for a little while at least. If we do this, the body tension will be reduced and we will feel more relaxed.

Diet and Muscle Development

The amount of energy we have, the vitality we have, can be influenced by other factors such as diet. While the general subject of diet is beyond the scope of this book, there are some aspects of diet that merit attention since they affect muscle development.

The outline of the body can be influenced by diet. If we eat more than the body burns up in our daily activities, layers of fatty tissue may form producing a heavier outline. The muscles are affected by this condition. Layers of fat may form between the muscle fibers. Inevitably, the tonic condition of these muscles is affected.

Your physician can advise you on how to control your diet. There is, however, one aspect of diet and your shape that should be emphasized. The most severe diet that will do wonders in reducing your waistline may not, probably will not, produce the contours which your body naturally can have.

When muscles have been encased in fatty tissue, and these muscles have not been adequately used, the elimination of the fat reveals the poor condition of the muscles. Their sagging now becomes visible. You have seen thin people with bulging abdomens and poor figures. Only adequate, functional movement of the muscles can remedy this condition.

Athletics and Exercise

In order to keep the muscles in tonic condition, we can rely upon our normal activities of the day, walking, bending, stretching. We can do Movement Schemes, that is, use the body functionally on the basis of the science of anatomy and body mechanics, to assure that muscles are being used properly. We can do formal exercises calling for vigorous body movement. We can engage in sports and athletics. The test of any movement aimed at shaping the body is whether it is functional movement conforming to the natural needs of human beings.

Athletics and sports have many benefits for those who enjoy the sensation of directing their movements, frequently vigorous movements, toward an impersonal goal: the point in tennis, par in golf. Such activities divert the mind from usual thoughts of self and its problems, and therefore afford the mind and personality relaxation.

Athletics of the more vigorous kind stimulate the circulation. The muscles contract and relax rapidly, blood flows through the body quickly, intake of oxygen increases, energy is speedily generated and consumed, the exertion brings perspiration and subsequent fatigue.

There are three points about athletics and exercise that should be stressed in their relationship to the tonic development of muscles. (1) The health of the body must be such as to permit these intensive movements. Your physician is the best judge of how strenuous an exertion you should make, particularly what movements are suitable to the condition of your circulatory system. Older people often find athletics and exercise too strenuous.

Happily these are not essential for the health and shape of the body. For (2) athletics and exercise may or may not help the condition of the body. It depends on *how* the movements are done. The fact that the body is being moved vigorously is not enough.

If in athletics and exercise the movements are performed functionally and the right muscles are being used correctly, then these muscles will achieve tonic condition. There is, however, the danger that the intensiveness of movement will cause *overdevelopment* of muscles. This distorts the shape. With advancing age when the muscles are less used, they grow flabby and sag.

Furthermore, vigor and movement does not necessarily mean that all the muscles requiring movement are being used. It is doubtful, for example, that many sports require the leg to be raised sideways, or the trunk to be moved sideways. Yet these movements are essential to the development and maintenance of tonic condition in some muscles.

(3) In modern times of urban living, the demands upon the body are not great, and therefore the development of the body that vigorous movements bring is not essential to health. However, functional movement is essential. Each muscle thereby receives movement adequate to maintain it in tonic condition. Most muscles can be so maintained merely by the movements we do in the normal day's activities. Some muscles, however, cannot be reached in normal activities. For these, the appropriate Movement Schemes, as indicated in the following pages, offer a practical answer.

Part II

THE MOVEMENT
SCHEMES

A NOTE ON HOW TO USE
THE MOVEMENT SCHEMES

1. *Stand between mirrors.* If possible stand between two full-length mirrors when you do the Movement Schemes. Arrange the mirrors so that you can get a complete view of the front and the back. This makes it possible to view the action of the back muscles. You will be able to follow the progress in the improvement of your muscles. You will also be able to guide these muscles and correct wrong movements when necessary.

2. *Follow each step as given.* The Movement Schemes are presented in as clear a manner as possible. Each step has its own significance and, though it may seem repetitious at times, none should be skipped. The aim of the Schemes is to provide help or information for individual needs. Each step has a part to play in reaching the specific muscle or muscles aimed at.

3. *Strive for accuracy.* The objective of the Movement Schemes is to reach specific muscles and to maintain them in tonic condition. Be sure you know

the muscle you are after. Then do the movement *slowly*, conscious of the specific muscle involved and the function it performs. Follow the instructions on the use of the muscle carefully.

4. *Do the movements slowly.* A characteristic of these Movement Schemes is their slow tempo. This enables you to "think" while you act, to become aware of the specific muscles required for each motion, to find them and to use them correctly. While slow in tempo, the movements are by no means slow in showing results; it can almost be said, the slower the tempo, the faster and surer the benefits.

5. *Do them as mild movements.* Most of the movements are mild and can be done by everyone. Some are to be done in the seated position, so that weak, convalescent or older people may profit as well. It is effective to do many of the Movement Schemes while seated; in fact, it is surprising how profitable they can be, even when done in this fashion.

6. *Be patient.* Some of the Movement Schemes bring rapid results, others require a longer time. Remember, in some instances you may have been neglecting muscles for years. You cannot make up for this in an instant. But with patience, and care in following the instructions, you can enjoy the benefits indicated.

7. *Apply the movements.* To get the full benefit of the Movement Schemes apply them throughout the day in your normal activities, sitting, standing,

bending, walking. The instructions suggest how. In this way, the functional use of the body will eventually be sufficient to keep it in condition. Daily movements will then become a source of muscle improvement, increased circulation and vitality. Requiring less energy, they will be less fatiguing.

And now, begin. Refer back to the health inventory of your body that you took in Chapter 2. If this shows no serious problems, begin by doing Movement Scheme 1 the first day. Do Movement Scheme 2 the following day, and continue in this way through all the Movement Schemes, remembering always to apply the principles learned to your movements throughout the day.

If the self-test shows body faults that require attention, turn to the appropriate chapter and do the Movement Schemes described daily until the condition is eliminated ·or greatly improved. Then you are ready to do the Movement Schemes in turn from the beginning, as above.

When you have completed all the Movement Schemes you will have a sound knowledge of the important muscles in your body, their functions and how to keep them in tonic condition. Through these Movement Schemes, and daily application of them, you can correct your body faults, have a youthful-looking body, reduce nervous tension and increase your vitality. Now it's up to you.

4.

COMFORT FOR THE FEET

Movement Scheme 1: Toe-Raising

The Aim

This movement improves the shape of the foot, particularly the toes and the instep. It can eliminate such conditions as curled, clawed, crooked, uneven or overlapping toes. It can also reduce the discomfort of bunions. It is aimed at the stretcher muscles of the toes.

The toes are raised upward, then stretched and lowered.

The Steps

1. Stand in balance.
2. *Slowly*, with the muscles along the instep, raise all the toes straight upward.

> You are using the stretcher muscles of the toes to do this.
>
> Try to raise all toes at the same time, and to an equal distance.

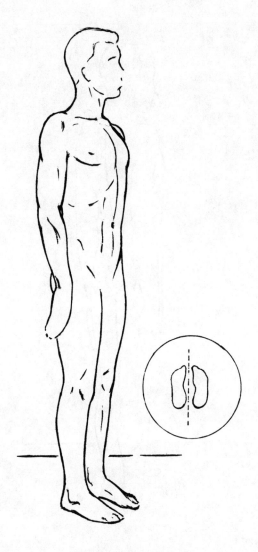

Stand in balance

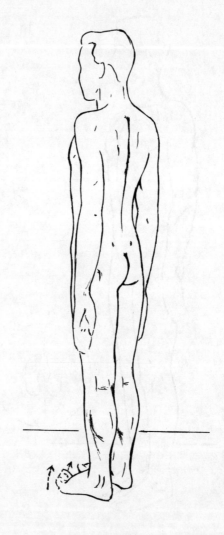

Raise the toes

You will be able to raise the big toe most readily; the others will require greater conscious effort, especially the little toe.

3. Hold all the toes raised a moment.

Become aware that now only the heel and the joints at the ball of the foot remain on the ground.

Sense also that the entire middle foot has been slightly raised, increasing the long arch of the foot.

4. *Slowly* lower all the toes and simultaneously stretch them out as far as possible.

Try to hold the toes as straight as possible, laying them down carefully.

5. When the toes have touched the ground, slowly release the tension of the muscles just used.

6. Do this Movement Scheme three times. Rest. Do it again three times.

The Explanation

This Movement Scheme calls into action the stretcher muscles of the toes. These are situated on the lower leg, between shinbone and calf muscles, and their actual muscle bulk is not visible. The tendons of the "toe-stretcher" muscles, however, can be seen along the instep of the foot.

In a normal foot they appear clearly as a decided

design of tendinous strings when the "toe-stretcher" muscles raise the toes.

In the daily activities of our civilized life we lack the freedom for natural foot-and-toe movements. Imprisoned in shoes which are often inadequately measured, walking on hard pavements or floors, constantly restrained, the foot is deprived of the normal use of its muscles, especially the muscles which move the toes. The toe movements which balance each other (clawing or stretching), thus keeping the toes in a straight and flexible condition, are restricted. Gradually the toe muscles become weak and the toes crooked, clawed or overlapping. The big toe joint sometimes develops a bunion. If the toe muscles are maintained in proper condition, crooked toes rarely develop.

This Movement Scheme will keep the stretcher muscles of the toes in tonic condition. If carefully and faithfully done, it will prevent or improve any distortions, and will ease the discomfort of bunions. It will establish an awareness of the ball-of-the-foot joints and keep them in flexible condition. This Movement Scheme is also helpful in adjusting the various small middle foot bones into a normally arched instep.

Movement Scheme 2: Heel-Raising

The Aim

This movement shapes the calf and slenderizes the ankle. It also improves the long arch of the foot. It is aimed at the calf muscles at the back of the lower leg.

You reach these muscles by raising the heels and shifting the body weight to the balls of the feet; then the heels are lowered.

The Steps

1. Stand in balance.
2. Distribute the body weight *evenly* on the heels and the balls of the feet.

   The ball of the foot is the area in back of the large toe and includes the big-toe joint.

3. With the calf muscles, *slowly* raise the heels off the ground. At the same time, transfer the body weight from the heels to the balls of the feet.

   Direct this transfer of weight along the *inner margin of the foot.*

Go only as far as the ball of the foot; avoid shifting the weight beyond the ball of the foot onto the toes.

Hold the buttocks and Adductor muscles (along the inner margin of the thighs) tight.

Keep the back erect throughout.

4. Now, *slowly* release the calf muscles and lower the heels to the ground.

Continue to press on the ball of each foot. Sense the transfer of body weight along the *inner* margin of the foot until it is again resting evenly distributed between the heel and the ball of each foot.

5. Slowly release the tension of the muscles just used, from the top downward.

6. Do this Movement Scheme three times. Rest. Do it again three times.

The Explanation

The muscles which raise the heel off the ground are the calf muscles. They are located at the back of the lower leg and form the Achilles tendon. This tendon is attached to the heel bone.

As the heel is being raised, the body weight is also raised and simultaneously transferred forward onto the ball of the foot, so that when the heel is up, the ball of the foot carries the entire weight of the body.

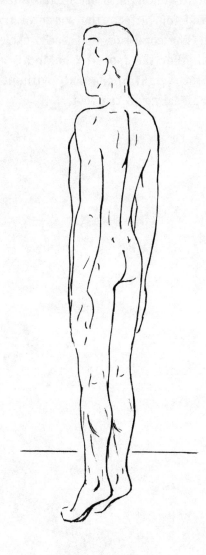

Raise the heels

Improper or inadequate use of the muscles of the lower leg and foot affects the shape of the calf and ankle joint. The condition of these muscles also determines whether the foot and ankle are capable of sustaining the weight of the body without causing a tired, aching feeling in the feet.

5.

REDUCE THE BUTTOCK AREA

Movement Scheme 3: Buttock Control

The Aim

This movement is aimed at the buttock muscles. It reduces the mass of the buttocks, tightening their outline.

The buttocks are drawn toward each other and then loosened.

The Steps

1. Stand in balance.
2. Place the right palm over the right buttock, and the left palm over the left buttock.
3. *Slowly* tensing the buttock muscles, draw the buttock halves toward each other. When they are drawn together as tightly as possible, hold them tight for a moment.

    Sense how the buttocks become firm against the palms.

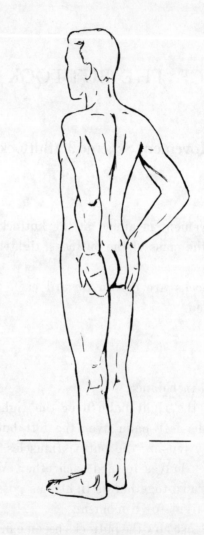

Place palms over buttocks

The buttock muscles can be tensed just like any other muscles of the body.

4. *Slowly* release the tension of the buttock muscles.

Sense under the palms that the buttocks become flabby as they are being relaxed. Keep in mind that the release of muscles should be as much under control as their contraction.

5. Do this Movement Scheme three times. Rest. Do it again three times.

The Explanation

The buttock muscles fulfill a definite purpose: they connect the legs with the upper part of the body. They play an important role in moving the trunk while walking or climbing stairs.

Other aspects of the function of the buttock muscles are discussed in Movement Scheme 4.

Movement Scheme 4: Buttock and Thigh Muscle Control

The Aim

This movement reduces the width of the buttocks by tightening them. It also improves the inner contour of the thighs. It is aimed at the buttock muscles and at the muscles on the inner margin of the thighs, called the Adductors.

The buttocks as well as the Adductor muscles are tightened simultaneously. Then they are released.

The Steps

1. Stand in balance.
2. *Slowly* draw the buttocks toward each other.
3. Simultaneously tighten the Adductor muscles along the inner margin of each thigh, drawing them toward each other.

> This will cause the inner margin of the thighs to become straighter.
>
> Notice that the buttocks become smaller and more rounded.

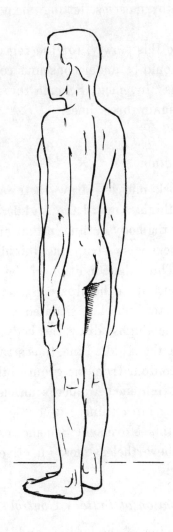

Tighten the Adductor muscles

4. *Slowly* release the tension of the buttock and Adductor muscles, letting them become loose again.

Do this slowly, for the release of muscles should be under conscious control.

5. Do this Movement Scheme three times. Rest. Do it again three times.

The Explanation

The buttock muscles draw their own mass and that of the thighs toward the Middle Line, thereby slenderizing the body outline in that area.

The buttocks also strap the thighbone into the hip socket. Thus, the condition of the buttocks also affects the outline of the hips.

The Adductor muscles, situated along the inner margin of the thighs, draw the body mass in this area closer to the Middle Line, thus straightening the inner thigh contour from the groin to the knee joint. The effect of tightened Adductor muscles will appear in a slenderer hip outline.

Although this Movement Scheme may seem very simple, it is nevertheless most effective.

Daily Application of Buttock Control

The tightening of the buttock and Adductor muscles should be practiced:

While rising from a seat.

While standing.

When reaching for something overhead.

Acquire the habit of tightening the buttocks in daily movements about the house or office. These movements will gradually become more graceful, light and attractive as these muscles are put into proper use.

Now that you have been introduced to the proper management of the buttock muscles, tightening them should become part of the Balanced Standing Position. This is the starting position for many of The Mensendieck Movement Schemes.

6.

FLATTEN THE ABDOMEN

Movement Scheme 5: Abdominal Control, Seated

The Aim

This movement eliminates the bulging abdomen. It helps maintain the abdominal organs in place. It also flattens the groin. It is aimed at the abdominal muscles which extend from the groin to the chest.

The abdomen is drawn in and upward, thus bending the trunk forward.

The Steps

1. Sit in balance:
   > On the sitting bone.
   > Near the front edge of the chair.
   > Feet flat on the ground, slightly apart and parallel.
   > Trunk and head upright.
   > Arms hanging at sides.

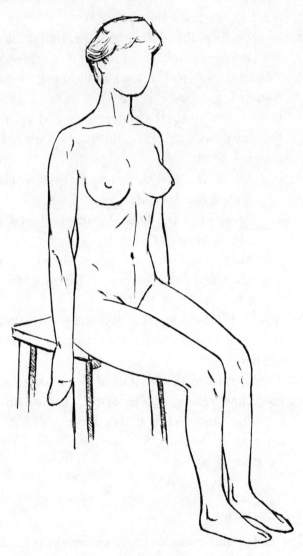

Sit in balance

2. Press onto the ball of each foot and simultaneously press upon the sitting bone.

3. *Slowly* draw the abdomen in, beginning at the lowest point near the groin, and continue upward to the navel, allowing the back to bend forward.

4. Continue to draw the abdomen in and up, past the navel, and to bring the trunk forward in a round bend.

   All of the abdomen from groin to chest should become flat.

   Press onto the ball of each foot and the sitting bone for support.

   Allow the arms to hang loosely at the sides and let them move forward as the trunk is being bent.

5. Now, still holding the abdomen flat, slowly raise the trunk until the back is straight again.

6. *Slowly* release the tension of the muscles just used, and release the pressure on the ball of each foot and on the sitting bone.

7. Do this Movement Scheme two times. Rest. Do it twice again.

The Explanation

The abdominal muscles have an important function to perform: they serve as a wall, preventing the contents of the abdomen, the intestines and the reproductive organs, from pushing forward.

The weight of these organs is greatest at the lowest section of the abdominal muscles, the part below the navel. Here the muscles tend to become weakest, and they no longer hold the contents of the abdomen properly. This becomes noticeable in an abdominal bulge.

In order to flatten the abdomen effectively, the tonic condition of the abdominal muscles must be restored.

Movement Scheme 6: Abdominal Control, Standing

The Aim

This movement also eliminates the bulging abdomen. It helps maintain the abdominal organs in their proper place. It flattens the groin. It is aimed at the abdominal muscles which extend from the groin to the chest.

The abdomen is drawn in and upward, thus bending the trunk forward. In addition, the buttock muscles are tightened.

The Steps

1. Stand in balance.
2. Draw the buttocks tightly together and, at the same time, draw tight the inner margin of each thigh.
3. Draw the buttocks slightly under.
4. At the same time, *slowly* draw the abdomen in and up, allowing the back to bend forward.

    Begin to draw the abdominal muscles in at

the lowest point near the groin, and continue upward until you reach the navel.

Press onto the ball of each foot.

Hold the buttocks tight and under.

5. Continue to draw the abdomen in and up past the navel, and bring the trunk forward in a round bend.

The abdomen, from groin to chest, should become flat.

Hold the legs straight.

Allow the arms to hang loosely at the sides and let them move forward as the trunk is being bent.

Bend as far as you can without straining.

6. Now, with the buttocks held tight and under, and the abdomen flat, slowly raise the trunk until the back is straight.

The arms hang at the sides again.

7. *Slowly* release the tension of the muscles just used, and ease the pressure on the ball of each foot.

8. Do this Movement Scheme two times. Rest. Do it twice again.

The Explanation

The abdominal muscles hold the contents of the abdomen in place. Their contraction bends the spine forward and downward.

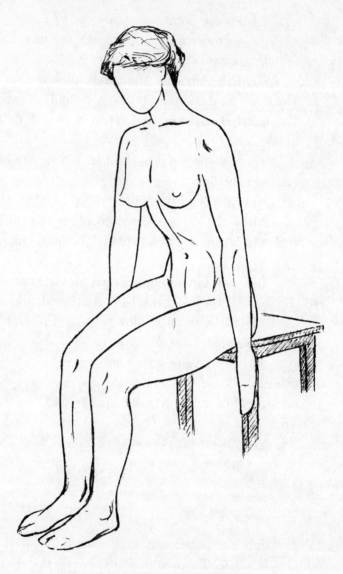

Draw the abdomen in

In the standing position, the buttocks assist the abdominal muscles in this action. They hold the pelvis steady, drawing it somewhat down in back, so that the abdomen can be flattened more effectively.

Daily Application

There are numerous opportunities in the course of the day when you can use the abdominal muscles:

> When seated, draw in the lower abdomen.
>
> When bending down to lace your shoes or to pick up an object from the floor, draw the abdomen in and upward.
>
> When reaching up for something overhead, tighten the abdominal muscles and the buttocks. (There is a tendency to push the abdomen out in the movement.)
>
> When lifting an object, hold the abdomen flat.

7.

STRENGTHEN THE BACK

Movement Scheme 7: The Back Stretch

The Aim

In addition to flattening the abdomen, this movement straightens the back and guards it against backache. It is aimed at the long back muscles which extend along the length of the back on both sides of the spine, and at the abdominal muscles.

After the trunk has been brought forward in a round bend, by drawing in the abdomen the long back muscles take over and raise the trunk again.

The Steps

1. Stand in balance.
2. Draw the buttocks tightly together.
3. Draw the buttocks slightly under.
4. At the same time, *slowly* draw the abdomen in and up, beginning at its lowest point near the groin and continuing to the navel.

5. Simultaneously, bring the trunk forward in a round bend, beginning at its lowest section above the buttocks, until the entire back is curved.

> Hold the buttocks in and under.
>
> Maintain the pressure on the ball of each foot.
>
> Allow the arms to hang loosely at the sides and let them move forward as the trunk is being bent.
>
> Throughout, keep the abdomen flat and the buttocks tight.
>
> Bend as far as you can without straining.
>
> (Toe-touching is not part of this Movement Scheme.)

6. Now, with the long back muscles *slowly* raise the trunk, gradually straightening the back.

> Begin with the lowest section of the back, i.e. the lumbar region.
>
> Straighten the back gradually, until it is again erect, including the neck and head.

7. *Slowly* release the tension of the muscles just used, and ease the pressure on the ball of each foot.

8. Do this Movement Scheme two times. Rest. Do it twice again.

The Explanation

The long back muscles have the task of holding the back erect. The bony arrangement of the back is a flexible one. It involves the spinal column, which extends along the center of the back from the pelvis to the head.

The spine consists of twenty-four small bones, the vertebrae, which are held together by means of ligaments, tendons and muscles, especially the long back muscles.

When the long back muscles are in tonic condition, they keep the back straight and hold the vertebrae in proper alignment. This Movement Scheme will contribute toward maintaining the long back muscles in tonic condition.

Movement Scheme 8: The Back Stretch, Completed

The Aim

This is one of the complete Movement Schemes to flatten the abdomen, strengthen the back and guard against backache. It is aimed at the abdominal muscles and at the long back muscles. Here the arms are included in the movement.

The arms are raised overhead. The abdomen is drawn in to bring the trunk forward in a round bend. The trunk is raised again by means of the long back muscles.

The Steps

1. Stand in balance.
2. Draw the buttocks tightly together.
3. Raise the arms overhead, palms forward, fingers pointing to the ceiling.
4. Draw the buttocks under and, simultaneously, *slowly* draw the abdomen in and up, beginning at its lowest point near the groin.
5. At the same time, begin to bend the trunk

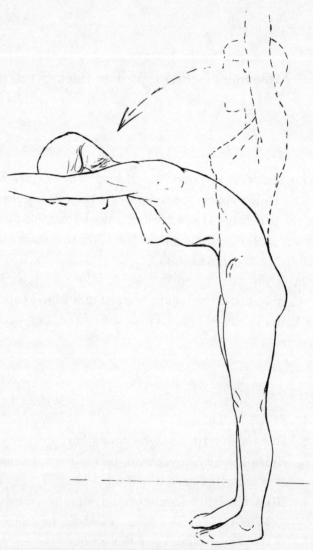

Bring trunk forward in a round bend

forward, beginning at its lowest section—the lumbar region—gradually curving the back in a round bend which includes the neck.

Stretch the vertebrae with the curve.

Keep the arms beside the ears as the trunk is being bent.

6. Continue to draw the abdomen in until it is flat up to the chest, simultaneously curving and stretching the back forward.

Hold the buttocks in and under.

Maintain the pressure on the ball of each foot.

Keep the arms at the ears as the trunk is bent. (Toe-touching is not part of the movement.)

7. Now, *slowly* begin to raise the trunk by means of the long back muscles.

Begin at the lowest part of the back, the lumbar region.

Think that you are returning each vertebra into place, straightening the spine up to the head.

The weight of the trunk is drawn upright by means of the long back muscles.

Throughout, keep the abdomen flat and the buttocks tight.

8. Slowly lower the arms to the sides of the body.

9. Slowly release the tension of the muscles just

used, and ease the pressure on the ball of each foot.

10. Do this Movement Scheme two times. Rest. Do it twice again.

The Explanation

The role played by the long back muscles in holding the vertebrae in proper alignment has been explained in the previous Movement Scheme. In fulfilling this action, the long back muscles sustain the weight of the trunk. They may be kept in tonic condition, thereby guarding the back against ache and pain, by means of this Movement Scheme.

8.

SQUARE THE SHOULDERS

Movement Scheme 9: Arm-Raising, Forward to Shoulder Height, Seated

The Aim

This movement will develop the shoulder and upper arm muscles in front, improving the lines of the upper arm and rounding it attractively. This movement will also prevent the appearance of hollows below the collar bone and will keep the shoulder joint in normal working condition. It is aimed at the forward arm-raising muscle, the front section of the Deltoid muscle.

Both arms are raised straight forward and up to shoulder height, and then lowered.

The Steps

1. Sit in balance.
2. Press onto the ball of each foot and onto the sitting bone.

3. Slowly turn both hands at the wrist until the palms face backward.

4. Slowly bend both hands backward at the wrist joint until the fingertips point backward.

5. With the upper arm muscle in front, *slowly* raise both arms forward and up to shoulder height.

> Be conscious of the action of the Front Deltoid muscle.
>
> Hold the elbows straight and the arms parallel.
>
> Keep the back and head erect.

6. *Slowly* raise both hands at the wrist joint until the fingertips point upward.

7. *Slowly* lower the arms in front by releasing the contraction of the Front Deltoid muscle until they are again at the sides of the body.

8. Slowly lower both hands at the wrist joint until the fingertips point downward.

9. Slowly release the tension of the muscles just used.

10. Do this Movement Scheme three times. Rest. Do it again three times.

The Explanation

This is the first of three Movement Schemes for arm-raising and lowering. Each will add a new phase until the entire movement is completed.

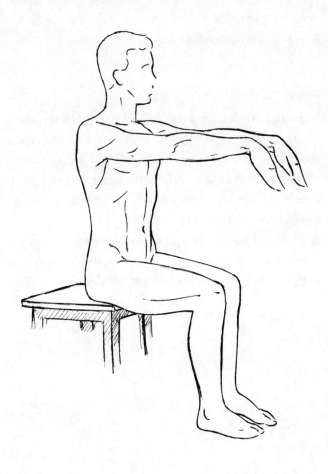

Raise arms forward to shoulder height

The "arm-raising" muscle is the Deltoid muscle, which covers the tip of the shoulder and extends to the upper arm across the shoulder joint. Its front section provides the power of raising the arm *forward* to shoulder height.

Daily Application

In the course of a day's activities numerous occasions occur for raising the arm forward and upward: combing the hair, shaving, putting on and taking off your hat or glasses, eating, smoking, carrying a tray, reaching for something, pointing at something and countless other activities.

Each of these frequent movements provides an occasion for using the Front Deltoid muscle, thus keeping it in perfect working condition.

Movement Scheme 10: Arm-Raising, Forward to the Vertical

The Aim

This movement will develop the shoulder and upper arm area in front. It will keep the shoulder joint in normal working condition, and will contribute toward relieving aches and pains in the shoulder region. It is aimed at the Front Deltoid muscle, and at other shoulder-arm muscles.

Both arms are raised straight forward and upward to the sides of the head, and then lowered in front.

The Steps

1. Stand in balance.
2. Slowly turn both hands at the wrist until the palms face backward.
3. Slowly bend both hands backward at the wrist joint until the fingertips point backward.
4. Using the Front Deltoid muscle, *slowly* raise both arms straight forward and up to shoulder height.

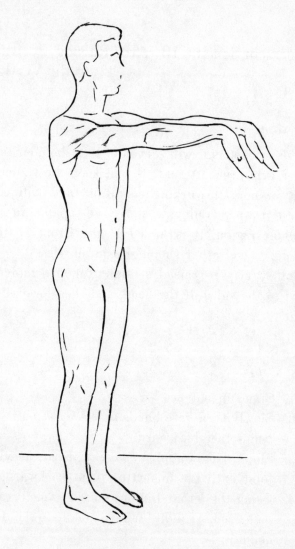

Arms forward and upward

Keep the arms straight and parallel.

Hold the trunk erect and the abdomen flat.

4. *Slowly* continue to lift the arms forward until they reach the sides of the head.

> Keep the hands bent at the wrist joint while raising the arms.
>
> Be careful to hold the shoulder tips down.
>
> Hold the arms straight and parallel.

5. Now raise both hands at the wrist joint until the fingertips point toward the ceiling.

6. Prepare to lower the arms by bending the hands backward at the wrist joint until the palms face the ceiling.

7. *Slowly* lower the arms in front as far as shoulder height.

> Keep the back erect, and abdomen held flat.
>
> Hold both arms straight and parallel.

8. Slowly continue to lower the arms until they are at the sides of the body.

9. Lower both hands at the wrist joint until the fingertips point to the ground.

10. Slowly release the tension of the muscles just used, from the top downward.

11. Do this Movement Scheme three times. Rest. Do it again three times.

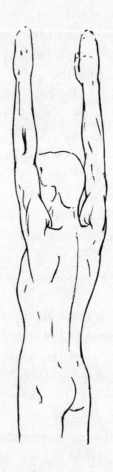

Arms at side of head

The Explanation

This is the second of three Movement Schemes for arm-raising and lowering. The forward-lifting movement of the arms makes use of other muscle groups at the shoulder-arm area. It thus helps to keep this region in tonic condition, attractively shaping the upper arms and shoulders.

It will also contribute towards keeping the shoulder joint in normal working condition, and will prevent or relieve aches and pains in the shoulder area.

Movement Scheme 11: The Rhomboideus Movement

The Aim

This movement will improve the outline of the shoulders, upper arms and back. It will flatten protruding shoulder blades. It also contributes toward a more slender waistline. It is aimed at muscles on the shoulder tip and the upper back, i.e. the shoulder blade muscles.

The arms are raised to the sides of the head, and then lowered sideways by means of the shoulder blade muscles.

The Steps

1. Stand in balance.
2. Slowly turn both hands at the wrist until the palms face backward.
3. Slowly bend both hands backward at the wrist joint until the fingertips point backward.
4. Using the Front Deltoid muscle, *slowly* raise both arms straight forward and up to shoulder height.

Keep the arms straight and parallel.

Hold the trunk erect.

5. *Slowly* continue to lift the arms forward until they reach the sides of the head.

> Keep the hands bent at the wrist joint while raising the arms.
>
> Be careful to hold the shoulder tips down.
>
> Hold the arms straight and parallel.

6. Now raise both hands at the wrist joint until the fingertips point toward the ceiling.

7. Prepare to lower the arms sideways by means of the shoulder blades.

8. *Slowly* lower the arms sideways, by drawing the shoulder blades together and thus lowering the arms to just below shoulder height.

> The shoulder blade muscles, the Rhomboideus and Trapezius, draw the shoulder blades together and flatten them. This shoulder blade movement draws the arms down sideways to below shoulder level.

9. With the muscles along the waistline, slowly continue to draw the arms down until they touch the sides of the body.

10. Slowly release the tension of the muscles just used, from the top downward.

11 Do this Movement Scheme three times. Rest. Do it again three times.

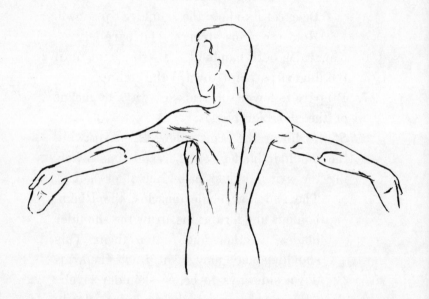

Lower arms sideways to below shoulder height

The Explanation

This is the third of the three Movement Schemes for arm-raising and lowering. Here the sideward lowering of the arms is indirectly accomplished by a shoulder blade movement.

The shoulder blades are triangularly shaped, flat bones, located on each side of the spine at the upper back. They form part of the shoulder joint in which the upper arm bone moves. Two muscle groups govern the position and movement of the shoulder blades: the Rhomboideus and Trapezius muscles. The Rhomboideus muscle extends from the spine to the edge of each shoulder blade. The Trapezius muscle covers most of the upper back and neck, extending from the spine across to each shoulder blade, to the shoulder tips, and upward along the back of the neck. The Rhomboideus is covered by the Trapezius muscle and thus cannot be seen. The Trapezius muscle, however, *can* be seen and its function observed.

The Trapezius and Rhomboideus muscles draw the shoulder blades toward the Middle Line, and simultaneously flatten them against the ribs. In approaching the Middle Line, the shoulder blades, in turn, draw the arms down to the sides.

This manner of lowering the arms sideways by means of the shoulder blade muscles flattens the upper back. This causes the chest to expand simultaneously, giving it a more rounded outline.

137

Movement Scheme 12: Arm-Raising, Backward

The Aim

This movement eliminates "round shoulders." It improves the shape of the upper arm and flattens the upper back. It is aimed at muscles across the upper back and arm; among others, the back section of the Deltoid muscle.

The arms are raised backward; then again lowered.

The Steps

1. Stand in balance.
2. Bend the fingers into a loose fist, thumb outside. Then bend the fists backward at the wrist joint.
3. From the back of the upper arm near the shoulder, *slowly* move both arms backward and upward as far as possible without losing the erect posture of the trunk.

   Use the back section of the Deltoid to raise the arms backward.

   Keep the back erect and the arms parallel.

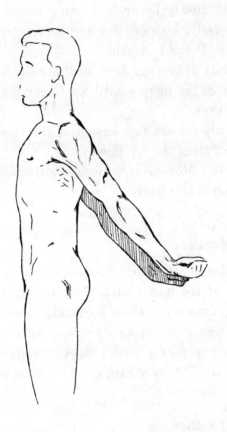

Arms backward and upward

Hold the abdomen flat, and the head erect. Press onto the ball of each foot and keep the buttocks tight.

4. Now, *slowly* lower both arms to the sides of the body, by releasing the contraction of the Back Deltoid muscle.

5. Slowly lower the fists at the wrist joint and stretch the fingers until the fingertips point to the ground.

6. Slowly release the tension of the muscles just used, from the top downward.

7. Do this Movement Scheme two times. Rest. Do it again two times.

The Explanation

This Movement Scheme tightens the muscles at the back of the upper arm, thereby improving its shape. It draws the shoulder blades together and flattens them, preventing "rounded shoulders." It holds the upper arm bone well within its shoulder socket, and effectively straightens the upper back.

Daily Application

Although the Back Deltoid raises the arm only half as high as the Front and Middle Deltoid muscles, it has nevertheless its own importance in the movements of everyday life. It makes it possible to raise

140

the arms to slip into sleeves, to reach into back pockets; it should also function when holding the hands clasped in back.

9.

INCREASE YOUR BREATHING CAPACITY

Movement Scheme 13: Breathing and Chest Expansion, Seated

The Aim

This movement improves breathing capacity and regulates the breathing rhythm. It is aimed at the proper use of the breathing muscles, i.e. the Intercostal muscles and the Diaphragm.

During inhalation the ribs are spread sideways, away from the Middle Line, by the action of these breathing muscles, and returned during exhalation to their original position.

The Steps

1. Sit in balance.
2. Place the hands lightly around the lower ribs on each side with fingertips pointing to the Middle Line. (The hands are being placed

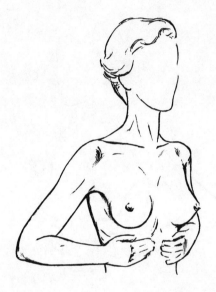

Place hands around lower ribs

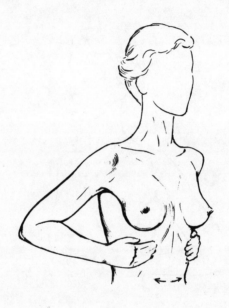

Chest muscles spread the ribs sideways

around the *lower* ribs where the spreading movement is greatest and may be felt most distinctly.)

3. Press the hands lightly against the ribs.
4. Now, very slowly inhale and spread the ribs *sideways,* away from the Middle Line.

   Feel under the lightly pressing hands that the ribs are slowly spreading sideways.

   This is produced by the action of the breathing muscles, the Intercostal muscles, which are situated between the ribs.

5. Now, very slowly exhale, gradually releasing the contraction of the Intercostal muscles, and let the ribs move in again toward the Middle Line.

   Feel under the lightly pressing hands that the ribs are moving in again.

6. Very slowly repeat the inhalation and the exhalation several times.

   Sense under the hands how the Intercostal muscles spread the ribs apart and sideways away from the Middle Line during inhalation.

   Sense how, during exhalation, the ribs move in again toward the Middle Line.

7. Repeat the breathing movement and become aware of the timing of inhalation and exhalation. Their timing should be of equal duration.

8. *Slowly* breathe in and mentally count the time it takes to spread the ribs sideways by means of the Intercostal muscles.

9. *Slowly* breathe out, and again mentally count the time it takes for the exhalation.

   Inhalation and exhalation should be alike in timing.

10. Repeat the inhalation and the exhalation until both are accomplished evenly and rhythmically.

11. Then lower the hands and let the arms hang at the sides. Repeat the breathing movement without the help of the touch.

    Become aware of the sideward motion of the ribs.

    Make sure that the timing of inhalation and exhalation is equal for both.

12. Do this Movement Scheme once. Rest. Do it once again.

Note: This consciously executed breathing movement should be done sparingly at first in order to avoid momentary dizziness. It may gradually be done more frequently.

The Explanation

Breathing involves two distinct movements of the ribs: during inhalation they expand apart and sideways; during exhalation they return toward the

Middle Line. Two muscle groups move the ribs during breathing: the Diaphragm and the Intercostal muscles. These are the main breathing muscles. They act together to expand the ribs sideways for the inhalation and their gradual release returns the ribs to their original position during exhalation.

The Diaphragm is situated between the chest and abdominal cavities. Since it is completely surrounded by the bony structure of the ribs, it cannot be felt by means of the touch as can the Intercostal muscles which are located between the ribs.

Since the action of the Diaphragm on the ribs during the breathing movement is the same as that of the Intercostal muscles, attention is drawn in this Movement Scheme only to the Intercostal muscles.

Proper use of these breathing muscles has a beneficial effect upon the body: it facilitates the rib movement and improves the posture of the chest. It also has a good effect on the outline of the abdomen: all undesirable forward pressure against the soft abdominal wall is avoided.

Scientific Side Line

Hundreds of years of controversy have gone into a scientific interpretation of the action of the breathing mechanism, especially that of the Intercostal muscles and the Diaphragm. It has, however, been established that the Intercostal muscles in conjunction with the Diaphragm bring about the breathing action.

Scientific data now available are quite sufficient to provide the necessary information concerning proper use of the breathing muscles.

Movement Scheme 14: Breathing and Movement

The Aim

This movement will improve the outline of the trunk or torso. It increases the breathing capacity, and reduces nervous tension.

It is aimed at adjusting breathing to movement: the breathing muscles and the Middle Deltoid muscle which raises the arm *sideways*.

The arms are raised sideways to shoulder height simultaneous with inhalation. Then they are lowered simultaneous with exhalation.

The Steps

1. Stand in balance.
2. Breathe in, using the Intercostal muscles and slowly spread the ribs sideways.
3. Breathe out, and simultaneously bend both hands inward at the wrist joint until the fingertips touch the sides of the thighs.
4. Breathe in, and simultaneously, *slowly*, raise both arms sideways to shoulder height.

    The Middle Deltoid muscle at the side of

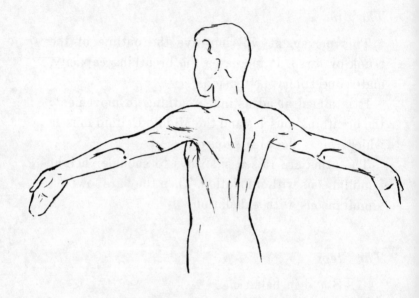

Raise arms sideways to shoulder height

the upper arm is raising the arm side-ways to shoulder height.

Try to time the rhythm of the breathing with that of lifting the arms and hands, so that both finish simultaneously.

5. *Slowly* breathe out, and at the same time stretch both hands at the wrist joint until the fingertips point sideways.

6. Now, *slowly* breathe in again and at the same time raise both hands at the wrist joint until the fingertips point upward.

7. Breathe out slowly, and carefully lower both arms to the sides of the body.

Take as long to breathe out as it takes to lower the arms.

Keep the hands bent upward.

8. Breathe in, again breathe out and simultaneously lower both hands until the fingers point to the ground.

9. Breathe in, again *slowly* breathe out, and simultaneously release the contraction of the muscles just used.

10. Do this Movement Scheme once. Rest. Do it once again.

The Explanation

There is a natural need within the body to adapt breathing properly to body movements.

When the arms are being raised, it is natural to accompany this movement with an inhalation; an arm-lowering motion calls for an exhalation.

Timing the breathing movement with the arm movement is equally important. It produces a certain rhythm within the body which has a quieting effect on the nervous system. It will make the movement more harmonious and pleasing.

Note: During Mensendieck lessons much importance is given the simultaneous execution of breathing and movement. To facilitate the comprehension of the Movement Schemes here, however, instructions for inhaling and exhaling are usually not included. How breathing can be fitted into the various Movement Schemes is demonstrated by a few examples which are given in Chapter 22.

The middle section of the Deltoid muscle raises the arm sideways to shoulder height. It extends from the shoulder tip at the side, over the shoulder joint to the upper arm bone. When brought into full use in raising or holding the arm sideways, the tonic condition of the Middle Deltoid muscle rounds the contour of the upper arm and shoulder at the side.

Daily Application

The Middle Deltoid muscle also has the function of holding the arm weight while the arm is hanging at the side. Certain daily movement habits—such as holding the arms akimbo; elbows bent and hands resting on hips; putting the hands into trouser or coat pockets; using arm rests or table tops which are too high—will relieve the Middle Deltoid muscle of its assigned task. If continued over a period of time, these indifferent movement habits will cause the Middle Deltoid to lose its rounded, shapely outline. In addition, the shoulder tip will be shoved upward, shortening the neckline or hunching the shoulders. Even the elbow joint will lose its pleasing roundness and become angular and pointed. To preserve the shape of shoulder and elbow joints, and the tonic condition of the Middle Deltoid muscle, the arm should hang freely at the side.

10.

SLENDERIZE THE WAISTLINE

Movement Scheme 15: Trunk Side Stretch, Seated

The Aim

This movement slenderizes the waistline. It is aimed at the side muscles of the trunk which form the waistline. They are the diagonal abdominal muscles.

By stretching one side of the trunk upward, the entire trunk is bent gradually over toward the opposite side. The waistline muscles of the stretching side are tensed.

The Steps

1. Sit in balance.
2. Raise both arms overhead, palms facing each other and fingertips touching.

   Stretch the elbows as much as possible and keep the arms in this position throughout.
3. *Slowly* stretch the trunk on the left side upward

154

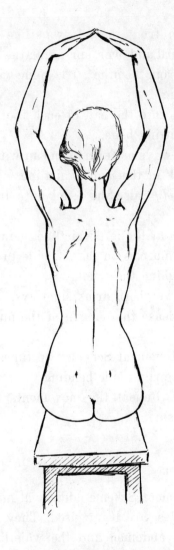

Arms overhead, fingers touching

and gradually curve it sideways toward the right.

> Begin from the left waistline to stretch upward and over, spreading the ribs apart, one from the other. The spine will curve to the right.
>
> Press into the ball of each foot, and onto the sitting bone.

4. Bend sideways as far as you can without causing a kink in the right waistline.

5. Now, *slowly* raise the trunk into the upright position.

> Begin at the left waistline, using the long back muscles on the left side to raise, and straighten the trunk.

6. Slowly lower both arms sideways.

7. Slowly release the tension of the muscles just used.

8. Do this Movement Scheme two times. Then do it from the right side bending the trunk to the left. Rest. Repeat the movements two times for each side.

The Explanation

In this Movement Scheme additional muscles, the waistline muscles, are being used. They affect the contour of the abdomen and the waistline. When these muscles are in tonic condition, they help to flatten the abdomen and narrow the waistline.

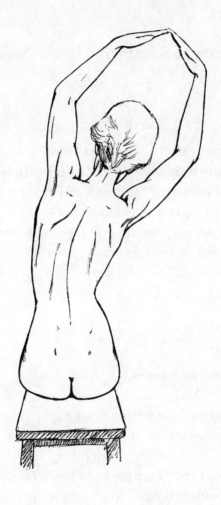

Bend sideways

Movement Scheme 16: Trunk Side Stretch, Standing

The Aim

This movement will slim the waistline, and will also improve the outline of the hips. It is aimed at the side muscles of the trunk which form the waistline, the diagonal abdominal muscles.

By stretching one side of the trunk upward, the entire trunk is bent gradually over to the opposite side. The waistline muscles of the stretching side are tensed.

The Steps

1. Stand in balance.
2. Raise both arms overhead, palms facing each other and fingertips touching.
   > Stretch the elbows and keep the arms in this position throughout.
3. Press firmly onto the ball of each foot and simultaneously tighten the buttock and Adductor muscles.
4. Now, on the left side, *slowly* stretch the trunk

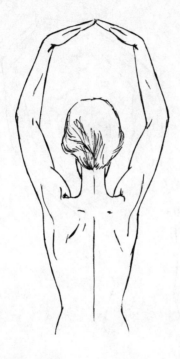

Arms overhead, fingers touching

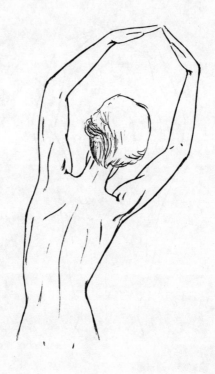

Bend sideways

upward and gradually curve it sideways toward the right.

Begin from the left waistline to stretch the trunk upward and over, spreading the ribs apart, one from the other. The spine will curve to the right.

Be careful to keep the body weight evenly distributed on the two legs.

Bend sideways only as far as you can without causing a kink over the right waistline.

5. *Slowly*, begin from the left waistline to raise the trunk to the upright position.

Use the long back muscles on the left to raise and straighten the trunk.

6. Slowly lower both arms sideways.

7. Slowly release the tension of the muscles just used.

8. Do this Movement Scheme two times. Then do it from the right side bending the trunk to the left. Rest. Repeat the movements two times for each side.

The Explanation

In this Movement Scheme mainly the waistline muscles are being used. When in tonic condition, these muscles help flatten the abdomen and slenderize the waistline.

In the standing position, the buttock and thigh muscles provide a firm base from which to stretch the side muscles and bend the trunk. In this manner, the benefit of the side-bending movement to the stretching waistline muscles becomes most effective. The overhead position of the arms offers added opportunity for increasing the flexibility of the entire spine in a sideward direction.

Since in the course of a day's activities we are seldom called upon to bend the trunk sideways, we thus fail to use these waistline muscles sufficiently to maintain a trim and slender outline, and keep the spine flexible in a sideward direction.

To rectify this lack, you might profitably do this Movement Scheme daily.

11.

END BACKACHE

Movement Scheme 17: Raising the Leg into
the Lumbar Region

The Aim

This movement helps to relieve fatigue and pains
in the lower back and sacroiliac region. It is aimed
at the muscles and joints of the lumbar region.

When contracted on one side only, the muscles of
the lumbar region raise this side slightly, thus raising the entire leg as well.

The Steps

1. Stand in balance.
2. Tighten the buttock and Adductor muscles.
3. Press into the ball of the right foot.
4. Now, with the lowest part of the long back
   muscles near the spine, *slowly* draw the right
   leg up into the lumbar region (the lowest part
   of the back). Raise the heel also.

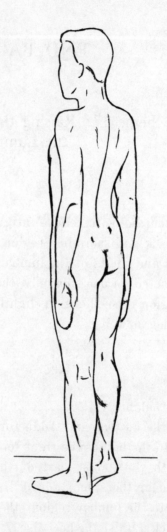

Drawing the leg into the Lumbar region

The ball of the right foot remains lightly touching the ground.

Keep the trunk erect.

Hold the buttock and Adductor muscles tight.

Realize that by this small movement the right pelvic half and the entire right leg have been raised straight upward.

5. Now, *slowly* release the muscle contractions of the right lumbar region, and carefully lower the leg until the heel touches the ground.

6. Slowly release the tension of the muscles just used.

7. Repeat this Movement Scheme two times. Then do it two times on the left side. Rest. Repeat it twice with each leg.

The Explanation

This Movement Scheme develops the muscles of the lower back area, i.e. the lumbar region. It renders the lower spine more flexible from side to side.

This conscious side-to-side motion of the lower spine, including the sacroiliac joint, helps to relieve tired, achy feelings across the lower back.

Movement Scheme 18: Raising the Leg into the Lumbar Region, with Weight Transfer

The Aim

This movement is also helpful in relieving fatigue and pains in the lower back and the sacroiliac region. It is aimed at the muscles and joints of the lumbar region.

Simultaneous with the raising of the leg, the weight of the trunk is shifted to the buttock and Adductor muscles of the standing leg.

The Steps

1. Stand in balance.
2. Tighten the buttock and Adductor muscles.
3. Press onto the ball of the right foot.
4. Slowly raise the right leg straight up into the lumbar region, thereby lifting the heel off the ground. The ball of the right foot remains lightly touching the ground.

   Use the lowest part of the long back muscles on the right side to raise the "dimple" and the right leg slightly.

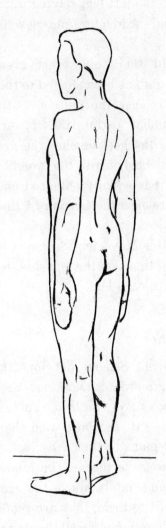

Raising the "dimple"

5. At the same time, transfer the weight of the trunk to the left leg, relying upon the left buttock and Adductor muscles to carry this weight.

   Hold the trunk erect even though the weight has been shifted to the standing leg.
6. Slowly release the muscle contraction in the right lumbar region, thus lowering the right leg until the heel touches the ground.
7. Simultaneously shift the weight of the trunk so that it is equally balanced on the two legs.
8. Slowly release the tension of the muscles just used.
9. Repeat this Movement Scheme two times. Then do it two times on the left side. Rest. Repeat it twice with each leg.

The Explanation

This Movement Scheme develops the muscles of the lumbar region which are seldom used in daily activities. It also curves the lower spine slightly sideways, increasing its flexibility and thereby preventing aches and pains in that area.

The five lowest vertebrae, the lumbar vertebrae, are located immediately above the sacrum. Having no ribs attached to them, they are readily flexible.

In the muscle relief of a well-developed lower back, a "dimple" is frequently visible on each side of the

168

spine in the center of the lower back. When the leg is raised into the lumbar region, the "dimple" on the corresponding side will also be raised slightly.

This Movement Scheme will be used again and again in other Movement Schemes. It is the preparatory movement for all subsequent leg movements.

Movement Scheme 19: Leg Pendulum, Backward

The Aim

This movement prevents and relieves pains in the area of the buttocks and the back of the thighs. It is aimed at tightening the buttock muscles, and contributes toward slenderizing the buttock area.

The leg is moved straight backward by means of the buttock muscle, then lowered again by releasing the contraction of the buttock muscle.

The Steps

1. Stand in balance.
2. Press onto the ball of the right foot.
3. *Slowly* draw the right leg up into the lumbar region, and simultaneously transfer the weight of the trunk over to the left leg.

   Rely on the right buttock and Adductor muscles to carry the weight.

   Hold the trunk upright, even though its weight has been shifted to the standing leg.

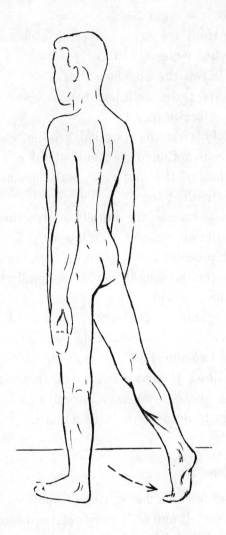

Draw the right leg backward

4. Now, with the right buttock muscle *slowly* move the right leg backward.

> Hold the trunk erect; consciously avoid hollowing the lower back.
>
> Keep the abdomen flat.
>
> Keep the right leg stretched while moving it backward.

5. *Slowly* lower the right leg, gradually releasing the contraction of the right buttock muscle, until the *ball* of the foot touches the ground beside the standing leg.

6. *Slowly* release the muscle contraction of the right lumbar region, and lower the leg until the heel touches the ground. At the same time, transfer the weight until it is equally balanced on the two legs.

7. Slowly release the muscles just used.

8. Repeat this Movement Scheme two times. Then do it two times with the left leg as the pendulum. Rest. Repeat it twice with each leg.

Note: If at first you have difficulty in balancing, hold lightly onto the back of a chair.

The Explanation

This Movement Scheme uses the buttock muscles directly, thus slimming the area of the buttocks, including the back of the thigh.

When you are seated, the lower spine, the buttocks

and the back of the thighs undergo constant pressure from the weight of the trunk against the chair. If continued over a long period of time, the buttock and lower back muscles become tired and irritated. Aches and pains may develop. This Movement Scheme will greatly improve the muscle tone and circulation in this region.

Since daily activities do not include the raising of the leg backward, this Movement Scheme should be done daily between mirrors. This will keep the buttock and back thigh area in normal condition.

12.

REDUCE THE THIGHS AND ABDOMEN

Movement Scheme 20: Leg Pendulum, Forward

The Aim

This movement improves the shape of the thigh in front. It contributes to a flattened abdomen, and benefits the lower back. It increases the forward movability of the leg in the hip socket. It is aimed at the muscles at the uppermost part of the thigh in front.

You raise the leg and move it forward in a straight line. It is then lowered to the starting position.

The Steps

1. Stand in balance.
2. Press onto the ball of the left foot.
3. *Slowly* draw the left leg up into the lumbar region, transferring the weight of the trunk onto the right leg.

Rely on the right buttock and Adductor muscles to carry the weight.

Become aware of this transfer of weight.

Hold the trunk erect.

4. Now, from the top of the thigh in front, *slowly* raise the left leg forward and up, at the same time drawing the lower abdomen in.

Be conscious of raising the leg by means of the front thigh muscles near the groin.

Hold the trunk erect.

Keep the left leg stretched and point the ball of the foot downward.

5. *Slowly* lower the left leg, gradually releasing the contraction of the muscles in front of the thigh, until the ball of the foot touches the ground.

6. *Slowly* release the muscle contraction in the left lumbar region, and lower the left leg until the heel touches the ground. At the same time, transfer the weight until it is equally distributed upon both legs.

7. Slowly release the tension of the muscles just used.

8. Repeat this Movement Scheme two times. Then do it two times with the right leg as the pendulum. Rest. Repeat it twice with each leg.

Note: If at first you have difficulty in balancing, hold lightly onto the back of a chair.

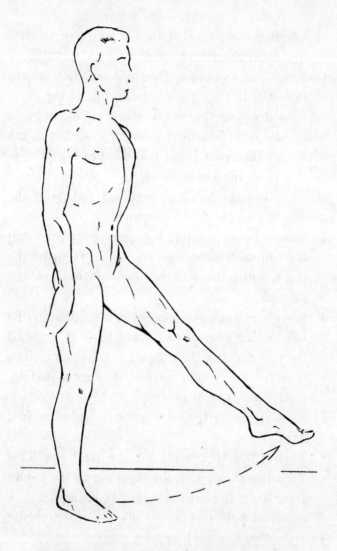

The upper thigh muscles raise the leg forward

The Explanation

The muscles of the thigh in front help to raise the leg forward. These muscles may become flabby and weak through insufficient use. This Movement Scheme will maintain the front thigh muscles in tonic condition. It will also reduce heavy thighs. The straighter the leg is being held during its forward motion, the greater will be the benefit for the thigh muscles in front.

This Movement Scheme points out the proper starting point for the forward lifting motion of the leg while walking: from the groin, with a flat lower abdomen. Such a forward swing of the legs renders the gait more youthful and graceful.

Movement Scheme 21: Leg Pendulum, Forward and Backward

The Aim

This movement improves the shape of the thighs, as well as the outline of the abdomen and buttocks. It also strengthens the lower back. It is aimed at the muscles at the uppermost part of the thigh in front, and at the buttock muscles.

The leg is moved forward, then backward.

The Steps

1. Stand in balance.
2. Press onto the ball of the right foot.
3. *Slowly* draw the right leg up into the lumbar region. Simultaneously transfer the weight of the trunk onto the left leg.

    Rely on the left buttock and Adductor muscles to carry the weight.

    Hold the trunk straight.
4. Now, *slowly* raise the right leg forward and up. At the same time draw the lower abdomen in.

    Hold the trunk erect.

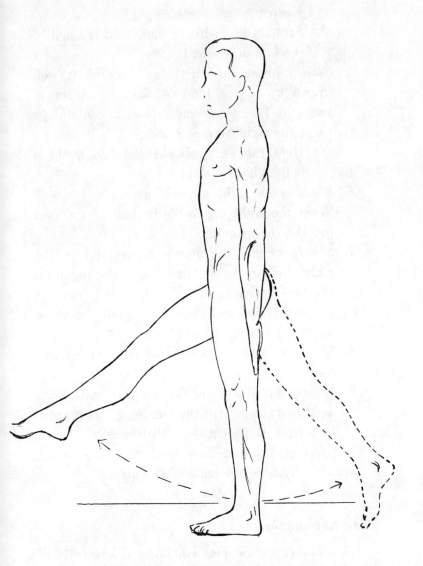

Leg Pendulum forward and backward

Keep the left leg straight.

Stretch the right leg and point the ball of the foot downward.

5. *Slowly* lower the right leg, keeping it well drawn up in the lumbar region, and slowly swing it backward and upward, consciously using the right buttock muscle.

Hold the left buttocks tight to avoid a hollow back.

6. Release the right buttock muscle and *slowly* lower the right leg until the ball of the foot touches the ground.

7. *Slowly* release the muscle contraction in the right lumbar region, and lower the leg until the heel touches the ground. Simultaneously transfer the weight until it is equally balanced on the two legs.

8. Slowly release the tension of the muscles just used.

9. Repeat this Movement Scheme two times. Then do it two times with the left leg as the pendulum. Rest. Repeat it twice with each leg.

Note: If at first you have difficulty in balancing, hold lightly onto the back of a chair.

The Explanation

This Movement Scheme combines the benefits of the leg pendulum, forward and backward. The forward movement reaches the muscles of the thigh in front; the backward movement uses the buttocks and the thigh muscles in back.

13.

SCULPTURE THE CHEST

Movement Scheme 22: Breast Muscle Control, at Shoulder Level, Seated

The Aim

This movement shapes the chest. It tightens the breast muscle, thereby raising the bosom. It is aimed at the breast muscle, the Pectoralis.

The arms are raised sideways to shoulder level, and moved toward each other until the hands touch.

The Steps

1. Sit in balance.
2. Raise the left arm sideways to shoulder level.
3. Place the right hand flat on the left chest above the breast, so that the fingertips are touching the tip of the left shoulder.
4. Consciously, with the muscle underneath the right hand, *slowly* move the left arm frontward.

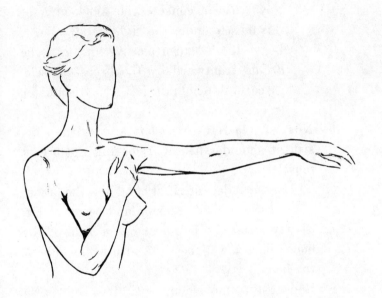

Hand on breast muscle

LOOK BETTER, FEEL BETTER

Sense how the muscle under the hand thickens slightly. This is the contraction of the breast muscle, the Pectoralis.

Keep the left arm straight, and at shoulder level.

5. Continue to move the left arm frontward with the Pectoralis muscle.

Now sense a considerable thickening of this muscle under the right hand.

Leave the left arm passive and let it be *drawn* frontward by the breast muscle.

Be careful to hold the left arm at shoulder level.

6. Now, *slowly* return the left arm to the side, still at shoulder height, releasing the breast muscle.

Sense under the right hand how the breast muscle loses its tension and becomes flat.

7. Slowly lower the left arm to the side of the body. Then lower the right arm to the side of the body.

8. Repeat this movement with the right arm going frontward. Rest.

9. Now, *slowly* raise both arms sideways to shoulder height.

Consciously lift the arms by means of the Middle Deltoid muscles at the side of the upper arm.

Keep the back erect.

10. *Slowly* move both arms frontward, consciously using the Pectoralis muscle on each side, until the hands touch at the Middle Line.

   Keep the straight arms at shoulder level.

11. *Slowly*, consciously using the shoulder blade muscles, draw the arms back to the sides until the fingers are again pointing sideward.

   Sense that the shoulder blade muscles have drawn the arms sideward.

   Keep both arms at shoulder height.

12. Slowly lower both arms to the sides of the body.

13. Slowly release the tension of the muscles just used.

14. Repeat this movement two times. Rest. Do it again two times.

The Explanation

This Movement Scheme is designed to keep the breast muscle, the Pectoralis, in tonic condition. The Pectoralis covers the upper chest, extending on each side from the Middle Line across the ribs to the upper arm. Its tonic condition keeps the bosom high, the upper chest rounded and attractive.

When the arms are held at shoulder height in this Movement Scheme, the horizontal fibers of the Pectoralis are mainly being used.

185

Movement Scheme 23: Breast Muscle Control, in the Diagonal

The Aim

This movement also shapes the chest. It tightens the breast muscle, thereby raising the bosom. It is aimed at the Pectoralis muscle.

The arms are raised to the diagonal position above shoulder level, and then moved toward each other until the hands touch.

The Steps

1. Stand in balance.
2. Raise both arms sideways and up to the diagonal position above shoulder height.

   Consciously use the Middle Deltoid muscle at the side of the upper arm to raise the arms sideways.

   Keep the back straight and the abdomen flat.
3. Now, with the upper section of the breast muscle, *slowly* begin to draw both arms frontward toward the Middle Line.

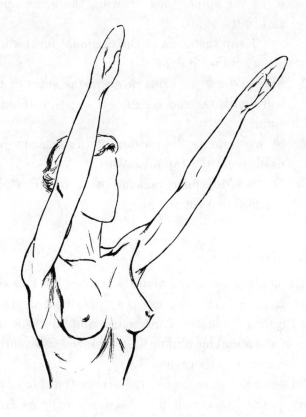

Breast muscle drawing the arms forward

Think that both arms are moving toward the cheeks.

Keep the back and the head straight.

4. *Slowly*, draw the shoulder blades together toward the spine, thus drawing the arms apart and to the sides.

Keep the arms at the diagonal level above shoulder height.

5. *Slowly* draw the arms down to the sides of the body with the muscle of the waistline (Latissimus).

6. Slowly release the tension of the muscles just used, from the top downward.

7. Do this Movement Scheme two times. Rest. Do it again two times.

The Explanation

By holding the arms above shoulder level in this Movement Scheme, you use the uppermost fibers of the Pectoralis muscle. Thus, a firm and youthful outline of the shoulder and neck is achieved, preventing the breasts from sagging.

The muscle which lowers the arm to the side of the body is the Latissimus muscle, which extends from the pelvis, across the lower back and along the waistline to the upper arm bone.

Using the Latissimus muscle for the sideward lowering of the arm maintains this muscle in tonic condition and helps to keep the waistline firm and slender. The Latissimus muscle can be regarded as "nature's corset."

14.

ABOLISH DOUBLE CHIN

Movement Scheme 24: Neck Forward Bend

The Aim

This movement beautifies the outline of the neck, eliminating a tendency toward "double chin." It is aimed at the muscles in back of the neck.

The head is bent forward in a round bend of the neck; then it is raised again.

The Steps

1. Sit in balance.
2. Press onto the ball of each foot, and onto the sitting bone.
3. Now, from the small of the back (lumbar region) with the long back muscles, carefully stretch the entire spine upward as tall as possible.
4. At the same time, slowly shove the chin slightly forward until it is being held at right angles to the front of the neck.

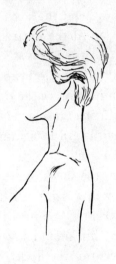

Chin forward, head erect

Feel as though the entire spine were stretching up to the "crown" of the head.

5. Draw the shoulder blades together and let the arms hang at the sides.

6. *Slowly*, from the base of the neck, begin to stretch and bend the neck forward and dov.n.

Feel the stretch from the base of the neck into the forehead.

7. Continue to bend the neck and head forward and down, until the entire length of the neck is curved forward.

Avoid tilting the head to one side.

8. Now, from just above the tightly held shoulder blades, with the muscles along the back of the neck, *slowly* begin to straighten the neck and to raise the head.

9. Straighten the neck, vertebra by vertebra, from below upward, until the entire neck column is straight again with the head well poised. The chin should now form a right angle with the front of the neck.

10. Slowly release the tension of the muscles just used, from the top downward.

11. Do this Movement Scheme two times. Rest. Do it again two times.

The Explanation

The head is balanced upon the vertebrae of the neck. The seven neck vertebrae form a continuation

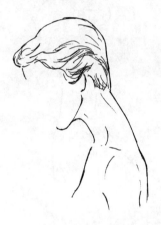

Round forward bend of the neck

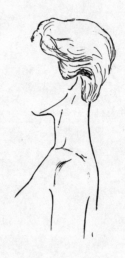

The neck column is straight and the chin forms a right angle with the neck

of the spinal column. The neck is held erect by muscles in the back of the neck.

The position of the head and the contour of the neck depend upon the condition of these "back of the neck" muscles. When in tonic condition from proper and adequate use, the "back of the neck" muscles hold the neck column erect and balance the head in a pleasing manner.

This proper use of the "back of the neck" muscles will prevent a double chin and will keep the neck outline slender. Do this Movement Scheme regularly if you wish to overcome defects in your neckline. Thereafter rely on correct movement of the head through using the back of the neck muscles as described in this Movement Scheme.

Movement Scheme 25: Neck Sideward Bend

The Aim

This movement improves the neck outline at the side toward the jawbone. It also maintains the flexibility of the neck column, and relieves tension in the back of the neck. It is aimed at muscles in back and along the sides of the neck.

The neck is stretched and the head bent sideward; then neck and head are raised again.

The Steps

1. Sit in balance.
2. Press onto the ball of each foot, and onto the sitting bone.
3. Now, from the small of the back (lumbar region) with the long back muscles, carefully stretch the entire spine upward as tall as possible.
4. At the same time, slowly move the chin slightly forward until it is held at right angles to the front of the neck.

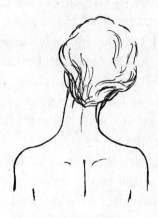

Incline the head toward the right shoulder

> Feel as though the entire spine were stretching up to the "crown" of the head.

5. Draw the shoulder blades tightly together and let the arms hang at the sides.

6. Now, *slowly* stretch the neck on the left and raise the left ear, thus slightly inclining the head toward the right shoulder.

> Use the muscles in back of the neck on the left to stretch the neck upward and to bend the head to the right.

> Hold the shoulder blades well together.

7. Then, with the "back of the neck" muscles on the left, *slowly* straighten the neck and raise the head to the upright position.

> The entire neck column should now be erect again.

8. Slowly release the tension of the muscles just used, from the top downward.

9 Do this Movement Scheme two times. Then do it two times, inclining the head to the left. Rest. Repeat these movements twice.

The Explanation

The "back of the neck" muscles hold the seven neck vertebrae erect, and safeguard their flexibility. This Movement Scheme improves the condition of the "back of the neck" muscles, and contributes toward a graceful sideward inclination of the head.

It also eliminates scrawny lines at the sides of the neck.

This Movement Scheme also maintains the flexibility of the neck column from side to side. It thus helps to relieve tension or pain along the base and sides of the neck.

15.

SLENDERIZE THE HIPS

Movement Scheme 26: Leg Pendulum Sideways

The Aim

This movement slenderizes the thigh along its outer side. It increases the movability of the thigh bone in the hip socket. It is aimed at the muscles along the outside of the thigh.

The leg is raised sideways and upward. Then it is lowered.

The Steps

1. Stand in balance.
2. Press onto the ball of the left foot.
3. *Slowly* raise the left leg into the lumbar region, thereby lifting the left heel off the floor, simultaneously transferring the weight of the trunk onto the right leg.

   Hold the trunk erect.
4. Now, *slowly* move the straight left leg directly

sideways, consciously by means of the outside muscles of the left thigh, as far as possible without strain.

Hold the trunk erect, although the weight has been shifted to the right leg.

Keep the right leg straight.

Keep the left leg stretched.

5. Then, with the Adductor muscles of the left *inner* thigh margin, *slowly* move the left leg down to its original position, with the *ball* of the foot lightly touching the ground.

6. *Slowly* release the tension of the muscles in the left lumbar region, thereby lowering the left leg until the heel touches the ground. Simultaneously, transfer the weight until it is equally balanced on the two legs.

7. Slowly release the tension of the muscles just used.

8. Repeat this Movement Scheme two times. Then do it two times with the right leg. Rest. Repeat it twice with each leg.

Note: If at first you have difficulty in balancing, hold lightly onto the back of a chair.

The Explanation

The muscles on the outside of the thigh (the Gluteus Medius) help to hold the thigh bone firmly in the hip socket. This gives shape to the hip area.

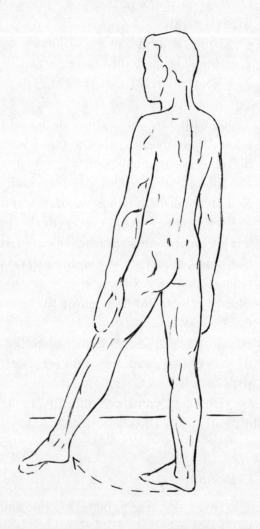

The side buttock muscles raise the leg sideways

From disuse these muscles may become weak and flabby. This condition becomes apparent as a heavy thigh, especially at its outline near the hip.

This Movement Scheme is designed to return the Gluteus Medius muscle to tonic condition. If it is done carefully and accurately, its slenderizing effect will soon become noticeable.

It is well to do this Movement Scheme daily at least twice with each leg. It will also have a beneficial effect upon the lower back.

Movement Scheme 27: Leg Quarter Circle, Back Combination

The Aim

This movement improves the shape of the buttocks, thighs and hips. It also strengthens the lower back. It is aimed at the buttock, thigh and lower back muscles.

These muscles are to be used by raising the leg backward, and from there moving it sideward.

The Steps

1. Stand in balance.
2. Press onto the ball of the left foot.
3. *Slowly* draw the left leg into the lumbar region, thereby lifting the heel off the floor. At the same time transfer the weight of the trunk onto the right leg.

   Keep the left leg stretched and the trunk erect.
4. With the left buttock muscle, *slowly* move the left leg backward and up, simultaneously drawing the lower abdomen in.

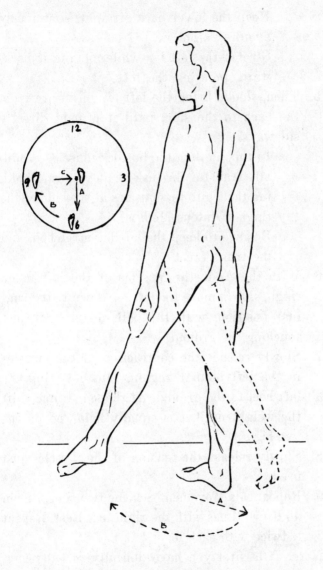

Move the leg backward; then bring it sideways in an arc

Keep the lower back straight, consciously avoiding a hollow.

Stretch the left leg while moving it backward, pointing the toes.

5. Then, *slowly* bring the left leg in an arc from the back to the side, until it is held directly sideways.

In this motion, the buttock muscles gradually transfer the task of moving and holding the leg to the muscles at the side of the thigh (Gluteus Medius).

Be sure to keep the left leg stretched, and the trunk erect.

6. With the Adductor muscles of the left inner thigh, *slowly* move the left leg down to its original position, with the ball of the foot just touching the ground.

7. Slowly release the contraction of the muscles in the left lumbar region, thus lowering the left heel to the ground. At the same time shift the weight until it is equally balanced on the two legs.

8. Slowly release the tension of the muscles just used.

9. Repeat this Movement Scheme two times. Then do it two times with the right leg. Rest. Repeat it twice with each leg.

Note: If at first you have difficulty in balancing, hold lightly onto the back of a chair.

The Explanation

This Movement Scheme reaches the buttocks, as well as the muscles of the outer side of the thigh. It helps to develop smaller and rounder buttocks. and slenderizes the outline of the thighs and buttocks. Also, it reaches the muscles of the lower back, thus averting possible aches and pains in that area.

Movement Scheme 28: Leg Quarter Circle, Front Combination

The Aim

This movement slims the thighs and the hips. It is aimed at the muscles at the top of the thigh, in front and along the side.

These muscles are to be used by raising the leg forward and upward, and then sideward.

The Steps

1. Stand in balance.
2. Press onto the ball of the left foot.
3. *Slowly* draw the left leg into the lumbar region, thereby lifting the heel off the floor. At the same time transfer the weight of the trunk onto the right leg.

    Hold the trunk erect.

    Keep both legs straight.
4. *Slowly* move the left leg forward and up, simultaneously drawing the lower abdomen in. Start near the groin and use the front thigh muscles to raise the leg.

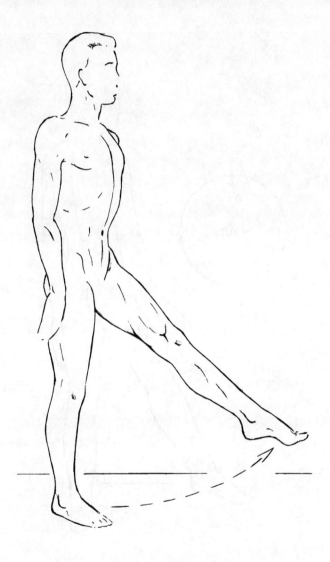

Raise the leg forward

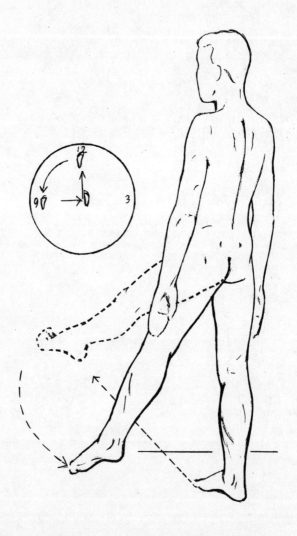

Raise the leg forward and bring it sideways in an arc

Hold the trunk erect.

Stretch the left leg and point the ball of the foot downward.

5. Then, *slowly* move the left leg in an arc from the front to the side, until it is being held directly sideways.

In this movement, the task of moving and holding the leg is transferred from the front thigh muscles to the muscles at the side of the thigh.

Be sure to keep the left leg stretched and the trunk erect.

6. With the Adductor muscles of the left inner thigh, *slowly* draw the left leg down to its original position, with the ball of the foot just touching the ground.

7. *Slowly* release the muscle contraction in the left lumbar region, allowing the left leg to be lowered until the heel touches the ground. Simultaneously, shift the weight until it is equally balanced on the two legs.

8. Slowly release the tension of the muscles just used.

9. Repeat this Movement Scheme two times. Then do it two times with the right leg. Rest. Repeat it twice with each leg.

Note: If at first you have difficulty in balancing, hold lightly onto the back of a chair.

The Explanation

This Movement Scheme reaches the muscles at the front and side of the thigh. It also tightens the lower abdominal muscles. If carefully done, these movements will improve the shape of the abdomen, thighs and hips. Also, drawing the leg up into the lumbar region serves to strengthen the lower back.

16.

SCULPTURE THE UPPER BACK

Movement Scheme 29: Shoulder Blade Shove, at Shoulder Level

The Aim

This movement flattens the upper back and reduces fatigue in that area. It is aimed at the shoulder blade muscles in the center of the upper back.

The arms are raised sideways to shoulder height, then the shoulder blades and arms are shoved away from the spine, then drawn in again.

The Steps

1. Stand in balance.
2. Bend both hands inward at the wrist joint until the fingertips touch the sides of the thighs.
3. *Slowly* raise both arms sideways to shoulder level.

> Use the Middle Deltoid muscle at the side of the upper arm to raise the arms sideways.

Hold the abdomen flat.

4. Form the hand into a loosely held fist with the thumb on the outside.

5. Now, *slowly* shove the shoulder blades and arms out, away from the Middle Line.

Think of the shoulder blade and arm as forming a unit.

Be sure to hold the arms straight and at shoulder height.

Hold the trunk erect, and abdomen flat.

6. Then, with the shoulder blade muscles in the center of the upper back, *slowly* draw the shoulder blades together toward the Middle Line.

Sense the shoulder blades being drawn in toward the center of the back.

Hold the abdomen flat.

Hold the arms straight and at shoulder height.

7. Open the fists and stretch the fingers until they point sideward.

8. Then bend both hands upward at the wrist joints until the fingers point to the ceiling.

9. *Slowly* lower the arms to the sides of the body, keeping the hands bent upward at the wrists.

Hold the shoulder blades tightly together.

10. *Slowly* lower both hands at the wrist joints until the fingertips point to the ground.

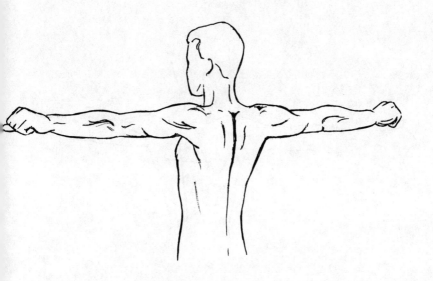

Arms at shoulder height

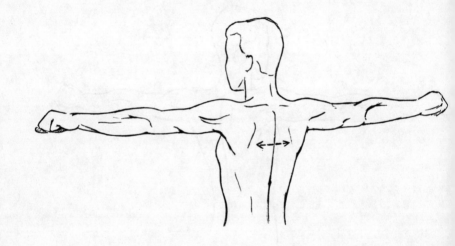

Shoulder blades apart

11. Slowly release the tension of the muscles just used, from the top downward.
12. Do this Movement Scheme twice. Rest. Do it two times again.

The Explanation

This Movement Scheme maintains the shoulder blade muscles, the Rhomboideus and Trapezius, in tonic condition. They then hold the shoulder blades together and flat against the ribs. This straightens the upper back and increases circulation in this area. The posture of the upper spine is improved. A rounded upper back may be straightened, or a stiff upper spine made more flexible.

Daily Application

Instead of being admonished, "Sit up straight!" a child should be told, "Draw the shoulder blades together!" Any postural improvement in the upper back should start at the shoulder blades with the shoulder blade muscles.

Holding the shoulder blades together can well be applied in daily activities:

When you are seated, it requires little extra effort to hold the shoulder blades together and flat.

When you are standing or walking, the same

217

principle applies. It is the "functional" manner of holding the upper back erect. It will provide lasting results in graceful carriage and a high chest.

Movement Scheme 30: Shoulder Blade Shove, Diagonal

The Aim

This movement also flattens and straightens the upper back, reducing fatigue in that area. It is aimed at the shoulder blade muscles in the center of the upper back, particularly at the *lower* section of the Trapezius muscle.

The arms are raised sideways to the diagonal position above shoulder level. Then the shoulder blades and arms are shoved away from the spine, then drawn in toward the Middle Line.

The Steps

1. Stand in balance.
2. Bend both hands inward at the wrist joints until the fingertips touch the sides of the thighs.
3. *Slowly* raise both arms sideways to the diagonal position above shoulder level.

    Use the Middle Deltoid muscle at the side of the upper arm to raise the arms sideways.

Keep the back erect, and the abdomen flat.

4. Form the hand into a loosely held fist with the thumb on the outside.

5 Now, *slowly* shove each shoulder blade and arm out diagonally, away from the Middle Line.

Think of the shoulder blade and arm as forming a unit.

Be ·sure to hold the arms straight.

Hold the trunk erect, and the abdomen flat.

6. Then, with the shoulder blade muscles in the center of the upper back, *slowly* draw the shoulder blades together toward the Middle Line.

Sense the shoulder blades being drawn in toward the center of the back.

Hold the arms straight and constantly in the diagonal position.

Hold the trunk erect.

7. Open the fists and stretch the fingers until they point sideward.

8. Then bend both hands upward at the wrist joints until the fingertips point to the ceiling.

9. *Slowly* lower the arms to the sides of the body.

Hold the shoulder blades tightly together.

Keep the hands bent upward at the wrist joints.

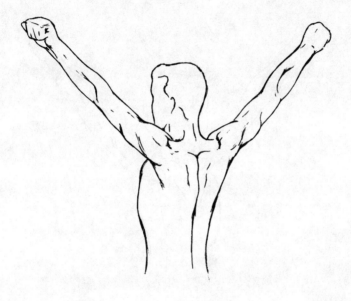

Arms in the diagonal position

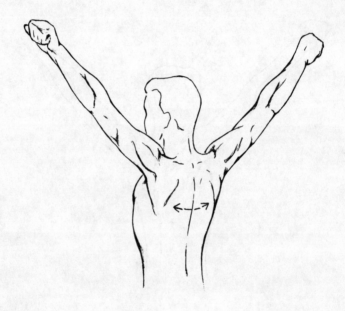

Shoulder blades apart

10. Slowly lower both hands at the wrist joints until the fingertips point to the ground.
11. Slowly release the tension of the muscles just used.
12. Do this Movement Scheme two times. Rest. Do it two times again.

The Explanation

This Movement Scheme also restores to tonic condition the Trapezius and Rhomboideus muscles, so that they may fulfill their function of holding the shoulder blades together and flat against the ribs. Thus, they will effectively straighten the upper back. This will ease fatigue and weakness between the shoulder blades.

Daily Application

In daily activities many forward movements of the arms are required. These tend to draw the shoulder blades apart, away from the Middle Line of the back. This may cause the upper back to become rounded. To maintain a straight posture of the upper back, the importance of drawing the shoulder blades together becomes evident. This Movement Scheme should be done attentively and frequently between mirrors.

17.

STRENGTHEN THE ANKLES AND FEET

Movement Scheme 31: Arch-Building Steps, Forward

The Aim

This movement strengthens weak ankles and improves flat feet. It shapes the lower legs and thighs. It is aimed at most of the muscles and joints of the legs.

The heels are raised, and small forward steps are taken on the ball of the foot with the legs held stiff and straight.

The Steps

1. Stretch a tape or string in a straight line across the floor. This will serve as a guide for keeping your steps *straight*.
2. Stand with one foot to the right and the other

224

to the left of the tape. Place each foot parallel to it.

3. Now, stand in balance.

4. Consciously using the calf muscles, *slowly* raise both heels off the ground until you are standing on the *ball* of each foot.

5. Then, carefully transfer the weight of the body to the right leg.

> The buttock and Adductor muscles carry this transferred weight.
>
> This frees the left leg so that it can now be brought forward in a small step.

6. From the top of the thigh, and without bending the knee, bring the left leg forward in a small step.

> Move the leg with the thigh muscles near the groin.
>
> Place the ball of the left foot straight forward on the left side of the tape, moving the foot parallel to the tape.
>
> Keep both heels raised, touching the ground only with the ball of the foot.
>
> Hold the knees and ankles stiff.

7. Then move the right leg forward in a small step in the same manner.

8. Now take several small steps.

> Move the feet parallel to the tape.
>
> Take even, small steps.
>
> Hold the knees stiff, and the heels raised.

225

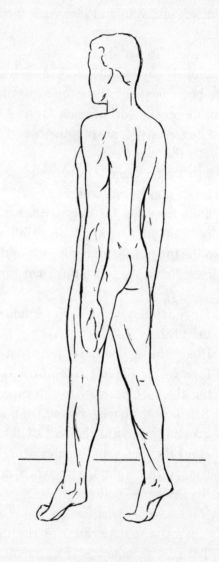

Small even steps forward on the ball of the foot

Think of your legs as being wooden sticks, only movable from the upper thigh near the groin.

Hold the trunk erect while stepping forward.

9. Stop. Bring both feet side by side with the ball of each foot parallel to the tape and the heels raised.

10. *Slowly* release the calf muscles and lower the heels.

Distribute the body weight *evenly* between the heel and the ball of the foot.

11. Slowly release the tension of the muscles just used, from the top downward.

12. Do this Movement Scheme two times. Rest. Do it again two times.

The Explanation

This Movement Scheme produces an awareness of the ball of the foot. Consciously used with each step, it builds a strong arch. It helps to overcome the harmful tendency to carry the weight of the body mainly on the heels.

This Movement Scheme develops the thigh, calf and foot muscles. It demonstrates the straight forward movement of each foot for correct walking.

227

Movement Scheme 32: Arch-Building Steps, Backward

The Aim

This movement slenderizes the lower leg. It also shapes the thigh and buttock muscles. It improves flat feet and weak ankles. It is aimed at most muscles and joints of the legs, particularly the calf muscles.

You raise the heels and take small steps backward on the ball of each foot, with the legs held stiff and straight.

The Steps

1. Stretch a tape or string in a straight line across the floor. This will serve as a guide for walking backward in a straight direction.
2. Stand with one foot to the right, and the other to the left, of the tape. Place each foot parallel to it.
3. Now, stand in balance.
4. With the calf muscles, *slowly* raise both heels off the ground until you are standing on the balls of the feet.

5. Carefully transfer the weight of the body to the right leg.

> The buttock and Adductor muscles should carry this transferred weight.
>
> This frees the left leg so that it can now be moved backward in a small step.

6. Now, with the left buttock muscles, move the left leg straight backward in a small step.

> Place the ball of the left foot straight backward on the left side of the tape, moving the foot parallel to the tape.
>
> Keep both heels raised; touch the ground only with the ball of the foot.
>
> Keep ankles and knees stiff.
>
> Hold the buttock and Adductor muscles tight.
>
> Keep the back and head erect.

7. Then, consciously by means of the buttock muscles, move the right leg in a small step backward.

8. Take several *small* backward steps.

> Move the feet parallel to the tape.
>
> Keep the heels raised and the knees stiff.
>
> Use the buttock muscles to move the legs backward.
>
> Hold the trunk and head erect.

9. Stop. Bring the feet side by side, parallel to the tape and the heels raised.

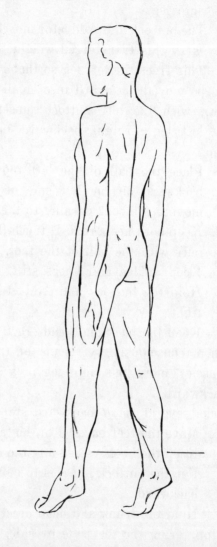

Small even steps backward on the ball of the foot

10. *Slowly* release the calf muscles and lower the heels.

Distribute the body weight evenly between the heels and the balls of the feet.

11. Slowly release the tension of the muscles just used, from the top downward.

12. Do this Movement Scheme two times. Rest. Do it again two times.

The Explanation

This Movement Scheme contributes toward strengthening all foot and lower leg muscles. It offers most effective help in relieving pains and aches in the lumbar region and along the back of the thighs.

It teaches the correct use of the buttock muscles in stepping backward and helps to keep this important muscle in tonic condition, tight and rounded.

18.

MOLD THE ARMS

Movement Scheme 33: Arm-Bending and Stretching

The Aim

This movement improves the shape of the arm. It rounds the upper arm, and straightens the elbow joint. It is aimed at the upper arm muscle which bends and stretches the elbow joint.

Holding the arms in the diagonal position above shoulder height, you bend and stretch them at the elbow.

The Steps

1. Stand in balance, palms facing thighs.
2. Bend both hands inward at the wrist joints until the fingertips touch the thighs.
3. *Slowly* raise both arms sideways and up to the diagonal position above shoulder level.

    Be conscious of using the Middle Deltoid, the muscle at the side of the shoulder tip.

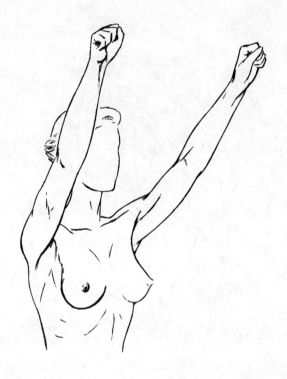

Arms forward and upward above shoulder height, hands
in a fist

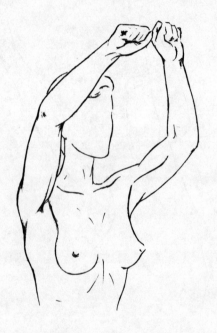

Elbows bent, fists meeting

Keep the weight well toward the ball of each foot.

Keep the buttocks tight, the back straight, and the shoulder tips down.

4. Straighten the hands until the fingertips point diagonally upward; then form the hands into fists, with thumbs outside.

5. With the "bender" muscles on the inside of the upper arm, *slowly* bend both elbows until the fists meet.

Keep the arms in the diagonal position throughout.

Avoid straining the neck muscles.

6. With the "stretcher" muscles on the back of the upper arm, *slowly* stretch the arms out again via the elbow joint until they are straight.

Check in the mirrors that the arms are straight.

Hold the shoulder tips down.

Keep the arms in the diagonal position throughout.

7. Open the fists, straighten the fingers, and then bend the hands backward at the wrist joints.

8. *Slowly* lower both arms sideways until they touch the sides of the body.

9. Slowly lower both hands at the wrist joints until the fingertips point downward.

10. *Slowly* and consciously release the tension of the muscles just used, from the top downward.

The Explanation

This Movement Scheme maintains the "bender" and "stretcher" muscles of the arms in tonic condition.

The "bender" muscles of the elbow joint (Biceps and others) are located on the inside of the upper arm, while its "stretcher" muscle (the *Triceps brachii*) extends along the back of the upper arm.

If you bend or stretch the arm haphazardly from the hand end, you give the elbow joint each time an indifferent pull or twist. This causes distortion, producing crooked or pointed elbows.

This Movement Scheme molds the front contour of the upper arm into attractive fullness, and stretches the back of the upper arm to firmness. It keeps the elbow joint straight and limber.

Movement Scheme 34: Arm Rotation, Outward and Inward

The Aim

This movement shapes the entire arm. It renders the arm muscles firm, and increases the flexibility of the arm joints. It is aimed at the muscles which rotate the shoulder, elbow and wrist joints.

While holding the arms in the diagonal position above shoulder height, you rotate them outward, then inward.

The Steps

1. Stand in balance, palms facing thighs.
2. Bend both hands inward at the wrist joints until the fingertips touch the thighs.
3. *Slowly* raise both arms sideways and up to the diagonal position above shoulder height.

   Be conscious of using the Middle Deltoid, the muscle at the side of the upper arm.

   Keep the weight well toward the ball of each foot.

Hold the buttocks tight, the back straight, and the shoulder tips down.

4. Straighten the hands until the fingertips point diagonally upward; then form the hands into fists, with thumbs outside.

5. Now, *slowly* rotate the arm outward, first in the shoulder joint, then in the elbow joint, and lastly in the wrist joint. The entire arm should now be turned so that the palm of the fist faces upward.

Keep the arms in the diagonal position throughout.

Keep the shoulder tips low and the neck free of tension.

Hold the buttocks tight and the abdomen in.

6. Now, *slowly* rotate the arms inward over the three joints, beginning with the shoulder joint, then the elbow joint, and lastly the wrist joint, until the palms of the fists face downward.

Keep the arms in the diagonal position.

Keep the shoulder tips low and the neck free of tension.

Hold the buttocks tight and the back straight.

7. Open the fists and straighten the fingers; then bend the hands backward at the wrist joints.

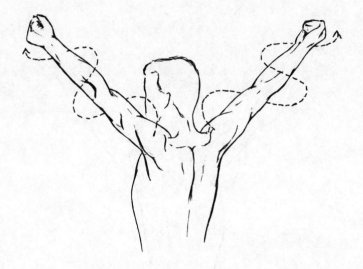

Rotate arms outward

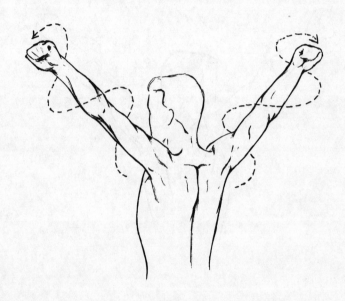

Rotate arms inward

8. *Slowly* lower both arms sideways until they touch the sides of the body.

9. Slowly lower both hands at the wrist joints until the fingertips point downward.

10. Slowly and consciously release the tension of the muscles just used, from the top downward.

11. Do this Movement Scheme two times. Rest. Do it again two times.

The Explanation

This Movement Scheme preserves the rotary muscles of the arms in tonic condition, keeping the contour of the entire arm firm and well rounded. It helps to keep the arm flexible in all its joints, preventing stiffness or pains in the arms.

Daily Application

You may hardly be aware that such rotating motions occur in daily activities. For example, shaking hands, opening doors, turning faucets, grasping objects of all kinds, or moving the arm forward when offering something—all of these require a complete or partial rotation of the arm joints. Even writing or drawing actually originates at the shoulder joint and includes a slight outward rotation of the upper arm down to the hand. Try to apply this Movement Scheme to these everyday actions.

241

19.

LIMBER THE KNEE JOINTS

Movement Scheme 35: Knee-Bending and Stretching

The Aim

This movement preserves the elasticity of the knee joint. It shapes the outline of the thighs and increases their firmness. It is aimed at the muscle groups in front and in back of the thigh.

The knees are bent gradually, without raising the heel; then straightened.

The Steps

1. Stand in balance.
2. Press toward the ball of each foot.
3. Draw the buttocks tight and under, and draw in the lower abdomen.
4. *Slowly* begin to bend both knees.
   Use the buttocks to bend the knees.
   Bend the knees slowly and resist a downward flop.
   Hold the trunk erect.

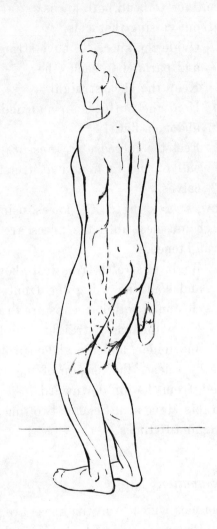

Begin to bend both knees

5. Continue to bend both knees as far as you can without raising the heels.

> Guide the knees to move straight forward and parallel to each other.
>
> Keep the back straight.
>
> Hold the buttocks in and under, and the abdomen flat.
>
> Feel the increase of pressure toward the ball of the foot, and a stretching in the calves.

6. Now, *slowly* stretch the knees, using the front thigh muscles, until the knees are completely straightened.

> Begin to stretch from just above the knee, and continue using the front thigh muscles until both kneecaps are drawn up.
>
> Keep the back straight, the buttocks in and under, and the abdomen flat.

7. Slowly release the tension of the muscles just used, from the top downward.

8. Do this Movement Scheme two times. Rest. Do it again two times.

The Explanation

The muscles which bend the knees are the bender muscles (Flexors), situated along the back of the thighs. The stretcher muscles of the knee (Extensors) are situated along the front of the thigh. To avoid too sudden a bend in the knee joint, the stretcher muscles should give in gradually to the action of the bender muscles, and vice versa when the knees are being straightened again.

If the knee-bending movement is done according to these mechanical laws, the movement becomes elastic. It may be stopped or continued at any point without losing power or elasticity.

This Movement Scheme thus increases the elasticity of the knee joints. It improves the thigh muscles, slenderizing their contour in front and in back.

Movement Scheme 36: The "Squat"

The Aim

This movement improves the shape of the thigh and increases the elasticity of the knee joint. It is aimed at the muscle groups along the front and the back of the thigh.

You bend the knees gradually while standing on the ball of the foot; then straighten them.

The Steps

1. Stand in balance.
2. With the calf muscles, *slowly* raise the heels. At the same time transfer the body weight along the inner margin to the ball of the foot.

   Hold the buttock and Adductor muscles tight.

   Keep the back erect throughout.
3. Press firmly onto the ball of each foot.
4. Now, draw the buttocks under and simultaneously draw in the lower abdomen.
5. *Slowly* begin to bend both knees.

246

Use the buttocks and the bender muscles in the back of the thighs to bend the knees.

Avoid a downward flop.

Hold the trunk straight.

Stand firmly on the *ball* of each foot.

6. *Slowly* continue to bend both knees.

Stop when the buttocks are still some distance away from the heels.

Hold the knees straight forward and parallel to each other.

Keep the back straight.

7. Now, press firmly onto the ball of each foot, and draw the buttocks under again.

8. *Slowly* stretch the knees, using the stretcher muscles along the front of the thigh.

Begin to stretch from just above the knees until the kneecap is pulled up and the knees completely straightened.

Keep the buttocks drawn under, and hold the back erect.

Keep the heels raised, balancing *only* on the ball of each foot.

9. *Slowly* release the calf muscles and gradually lower both heels.

Let the body weight travel along the *inner* margin of the foot until both heels have reached the ground. The body weight should now be evenly distributed between the ball and heel of each foot.

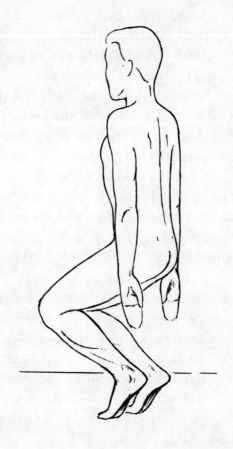

Bend the knees slowly

10. Slowly release the tension of the muscles just used, from the top downward.
11. Do this Movement Scheme two times. Rest. Do it again two times.

The Explanation

This Movement Scheme further increases the elasticity of the knee joints. Being executed on the small area, the ball of the foot, it becomes simultaneously a balancing exercise. During this "squatting" movement, the body weight is being lowered and then raised again while resting on the ball-of-the-foot joints. These act like a rocker, making constant adjustments to balance the body weight above them.

Simultaneously, similar adjustments must be made in all other joints; thus the benefit for all leg joints is increased, including especially those of the entire foot.

20.

SHAPE THE LEGS

Movement Scheme 37: The "Squat" in Step Position

The Aim

This movement shapes the contour of the thighs and calves, and improves the flexibility of the knee and ankle joints. It is aimed at the thigh and calf muscles.

While you stand on the ball of each foot, the knees are bent, and then stretched erect.

The Steps

1. Stand in balance.
2. *Slowly* raise the right leg, using the muscles of the lumbar region, thereby transferring the body weight to the left leg.
3. Bring the right leg forward in a small step; let only the ball of the foot touch the ground, with the heel raised.
4. Now, with the left calf muscle, *slowly* raise

the left heel, rising onto the ball of each foot.

Distribute the body weight evenly between the balls of the feet.

Hold the buttock and Adductor muscles tight.

Keep the trunk erect, and the legs straight.

5. Draw the buttocks under, and draw the lower abdomen in.

6. Now, *slowly* begin to bend both knees, using the buttocks and the bender muscles at the back of the thighs.

Hold the knees straight forward and keep them parallel to each other.

Hold the trunk erect and the abdomen in.

7. Now, pressing firmly onto the ball of each foot, *slowly* stretch the knees, using the stretcher muscles along the front of the thighs.

Begin to stretch from just above the knees, pulling the kneecap up until both knees are straightened.

Hold the back straight and the heels raised.

Keep the buttocks drawn under.

8. Shift the body weight gradually backward to the left leg and slowly lower the left heel.

9. Draw the right leg up, and move it backward until the ball of the right foot touches the ground beside the standing leg.

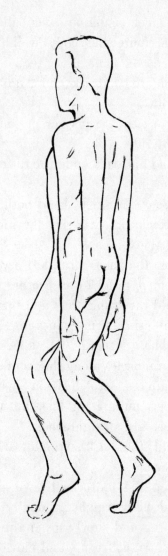

Bend the knees using the bender muscles

10. Now, lower the right leg until the heel touches the ground, at the same time transferring the weight of the body until it is evenly distributed on both legs.

11. Slowly release the tension of the muscles just used, from the top downward.

12. Do this Movement Scheme two times. Rest. Do it again two times.

The Explanation

This Movement Scheme offers the same benefits as the "Squat." It renders the knee joints more elastic and protects them from irritation or pain.

It also strengthens the feet and improves all thigh and lower leg muscles.

Movement Scheme 38: "Knee-Saw"

The Aim

This movement increases the elasticity of the knee joints. It contributes toward a youthful and graceful manner of walking. It is aimed at the muscles in the front and back of the thighs, as well as the calf muscles.

While in step-squatting position, the body weight is shifted from one leg to the other in a seesaw motion.

The Steps

1. Stand in balance.
2. *Slowly* raise the right leg in the lumbar region.
3. Bring the right leg forward in a small step. Let only the ball of the foot touch the ground, with the heel slightly raised.
4. With the left calf muscle *slowly* raise the left heel, thus rising onto the balls of both feet.

   Keep the trunk erect and the legs straight.

   Distribute the body weight evenly.
5. Draw the buttocks under, and draw the lower abdomen in.

6. Now, *slowly* bend both knees, using the buttocks and the bender muscles at the back of the thighs.

> Hold the knees straight forward and parallel to each other.

> Keep the trunk erect.

7. While in this squatting position, *slowly*, with the buttock muscles, move the weight of the trunk forward until it is being carried by the right leg.

> Keep the knees bent at the same angle and hold the buttocks at the same height from the ground.

8. Now, *slowly* shift the weight of the trunk backward until it rests mainly on the left leg.

> Keep the buttock and Adductor muscles tight.

> Hold the back straight.

9. Repeat this "seesaw" motion two times.

10. Press firmly onto the ball of each foot.

11. With the weight mainly sustained by the left leg, *slowly* stretch both knees erect, using the stretcher muscles along the front thigh, until both knees are straight again with the kneecaps drawn up.

> Keep the back straight and the heels raised.

12. *Slowly* lower the left heel, by releasing the contraction of the calf muscles.

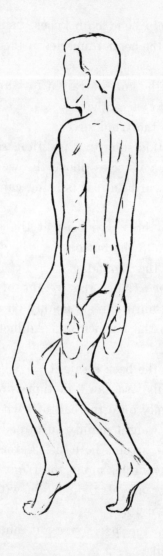

Shift the weight from one foot to the other

13. Draw the right leg up from the lumbar region, and move it back into place until the ball of the right foot is touching the ground.

14. Now lower the right leg from the lumbar region until the heel touches the ground. At the same time, transfer the weight of the body until it is evenly balanced on both legs.

15. Slowly release the tension of the muscles just used, from the top downward.

16. Do this Movement Scheme once. Rest. Do it once again.

The Explanation

This Movement Scheme is designed to increase the elasticity of all the leg joints, especially that of the knee joint. Thus, it contributes toward a youthful and elastic gait.

It is the basic movement in numerous daily activities: sitting, rising, kneeling, walking up and down stairs, and many others which require the bending and stretching of the knees. You have therefore many opportunities during the day to do this beneficial movement correctly.

21.

STRENGTHEN THE FEET

Movement Scheme 39: Jumping

The Aim

This movement strengthens the legs, particularly the calf muscles. It is aimed at the feet, calf and thigh muscles.

Short hops on the ball of the foot are executed with stiffly held legs.

The Steps

1. Stand in balance.
2. With the calf muscles *quickly* raise the heels and jump forward repeatedly in a series of little hops.

   > Hop in a straight line.
   > Land each time on the balls of the feet, without lowering the heels.
   > Hold the knee and ankle joints stiff.
   > Keep the back erect.

3. After hopping a number of times, stop. Re-

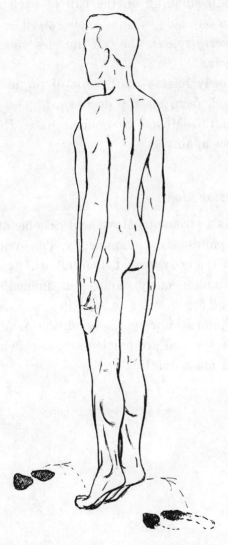

Short hops forward on the ball of the foot

main standing on the ball of each foot, with the feet side by side, heels raised.

4. *Slowly* release the calf muscles and lower the heels.

5. Slowly release the tension of the muscles just used, from the top downward.

6. Do this Movement Scheme once. Rest. Do it once again.

The Explanation

This is a strenuous Movement Scheme and should be done cautiously and sparingly. The sudden imposition of the body weight upon all stiff leg and foot joints simultaneously requires an immediate readiness of all leg muscles to sustain this shock. These sudden jumps improve the condition of all leg and foot muscles, and are particularly beneficial for the foot and ankle joints.

22.

COMBINED MOVEMENT SCHEMES

Movement Scheme 40: Arm-Raising and Breathing in Rhythm

The Aim

To shape the shoulders, upper arms and upper back, as well as the waistline.

The Steps

1. Stand in balance.
2. *Inhale* slowly. *Exhale* as you bend the hands backward at the wrist joints so that the finger-tips point backward.
3. *Inhale* and at the same time, with the Front Deltoid muscles at the shoulder tips in front, slowly raise both arms forward and upward to shoulder height. Stop and *exhale*.

   Hold the arms straight at the elbows.
   Keep the arms parallel.
   Maintain a straight flat back.

4. *Inhale* and, at the same time, slowly raise the arms forward and upward until the arms reach the side of the head at the ears.

    Be careful to hold the shoulder tips down. Hold the arms stretched, straight and parallel.

    Keep the hands bent at the wrists.

5. *Exhale* as you raise the hands at the wrists so that the fingertips point to the ceiling.

6. *Inhale* as you slant both hands sideways at the wrist toward the small finger so that the thumb points to the ceiling.

7. *Exhale* as you lower the arms sideways, using the shoulder blade muscles to draw the shoulder blades together and thereby bringing the arms down to slightly below shoulder height. Stop.

    Muscles near the nape of the neck and at the upper part of the back draw the shoulder blades together and flat. The shoulder blade movement draws the arms down sideways.

8. *Inhale.* Then *exhale* slowly as you use the muscles along the waistline to draw the arms down until they are touching the sides of the body.

9. Now slowly release the back and shoulder blade muscles, and other muscles, from the top down, to restore the body to the "relaxed" position.

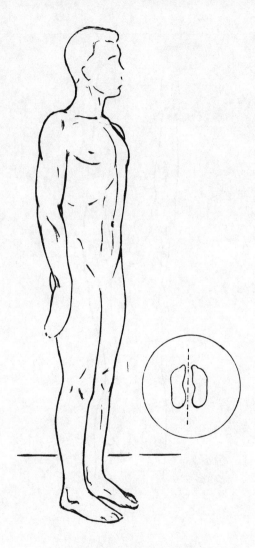

Stand in balance

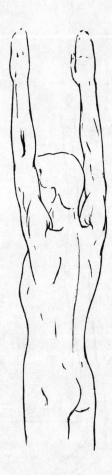

Arms at side of head

Movement Scheme 41 : Round Forward Trunk Bend Combined with Breathing

The Aim

To flatten the abdomen, strengthen the back and guard against backache.

The Steps

1. Stand in balance.
2. *Breathe in* slowly. *Breathe out* slowly as you bend the hands backward at the wrist joints so that the fingertips point backward.
3. *Breathe in* slowly and, simultaneously, with the Front Deltoid muscles at the shoulder tips in front, slowly raise both arms forward and upward to shoulder height. Stop and slowly *breathe out*.
4. *Breathe in* as you continue slowly to raise the arms forward and upward until the arms reach the sides of the head at the ears.
5. *Breathe out* as you bend the hands at the wrist joints so that the palms face the ceiling.

6. *Inhale.* Now, *exhale* as you draw the buttocks under, and simultaneously draw the abdomen in and up, beginning at the lowest point near the groin.

7. At the same time, bring the trunk forward in a round bend, beginning at its lowest section above the buttocks, until the entire back is curved forward.

8. Keep the arms along the sides of the head at the ears as the trunk bends.

9. Continue to *exhale* and complete drawing the abdomen in until it is flat. At the same time continue to bend the back as far forward as you can without straining.

> Hold the buttocks in and under.
>
> Maintain the pressure on the ball of the foot.
>
> Hold the arms along the ears as the trunk bends forward and down.
>
> Toe-touching is not part of this Movement Scheme.

10. *Breathe in* as you slowly raise the trunk with the long back muscles, gradually straightening the back.

> Begin at the lowest part of the back, the lumbar vertebrae region.
>
> You are drawing the weight of the trunk up into position by means of long back muscles.

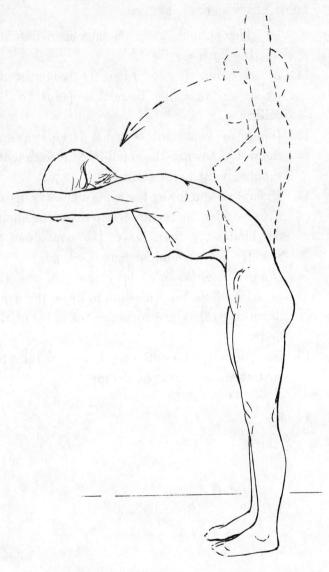

Trunk forward in a round bend

Throughout, keep the abdomen flat and the buttocks tight.

11. *Breathe out* as you raise the hands at the wrists so that the fingertips point to the ceiling.

12. *Inhale* as you slant both hands sideways at the wrists toward the small fingers so that the thumbs point to the ceiling.

13. *Exhale* as you lower the arms sideways, using the shoulder blade muscles to draw the shoulder blades together. Lower the arms down to slightly below shoulder height. Stop.

14. *Inhale*. Then *exhale* slowly as you use the muscles along the waistline to draw the arms down until they are touching the sides of the body.

15. Now, slowly release the tension of the muscles just used, beginning at the top.

Movement Scheme 42: Leg Pendulum Forward and Backward, Combined with Breathing

The Aim

To shape the thighs, abdomen and buttocks, as well as to strengthen the lower back.

The Steps

1. Stand in balance.
2. Press onto the ball of the right foot.
3. Simultaneously transfer the weight of the trunk onto the left leg, and *slowly* draw the right leg up into the lumbar region.

   Rely on the left buttock and Adductor muscles to carry the weight.

   Hold the trunk straight.
4. Inhale. Exhale *slowly* and simultaneously raise the right leg forward and up. At the same time draw the lower abdomen in.

   Hold the trunk erect.

   Keep the left leg straight.

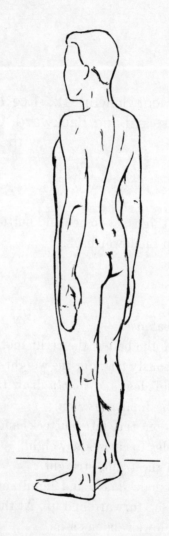

Drawing the leg into the Lumbar region

Stretch the right leg and point the ball of the foot downward.

5. Inhale. Exhale and at the same time *slowly* lower the right leg, keeping it well drawn up in the lumbar region, and slowly swing it backward and upward, consciously using the right buttock muscle.

    Hold the left buttock tight to avoid a hollow back.

6. Inhale. Exhale and simultaneously release the right buttock muscle and *slowly* lower the right leg until the ball of the foot touches the ground.

7. *Slowly* release the muscle contraction in the right lumbar region, and lower the right leg until the heel touches the ground. Simultaneously transfer the weight until it is equally balanced on the two legs.

8. Slowly release the tension of the muscles just used.

9. Repeat these movements standing on the right leg and raising the left one.

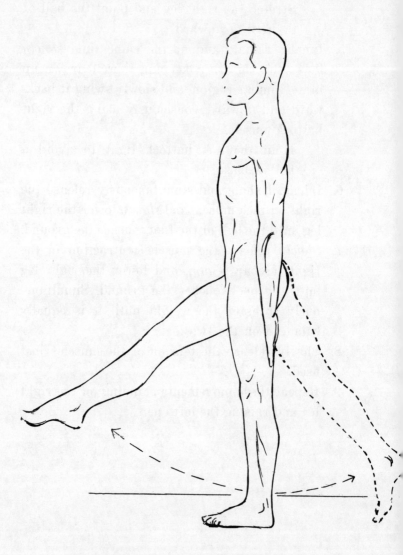

The leg pendulum forward and backward

Movement Scheme 43 : Trunk Side Stretch, Combined with Breathing

The Aim

To slenderize the waistline and flatten the abdomen.

The Steps

1. Stand in balance.
2. Raise both arms overhead, palms facing each other and fingertips touching.

   Stretch the elbows and keep the arms in this position throughout.
3. Press firmly onto the ball of each foot and simultaneously tighten the buttock and Adductor muscles.
4. Now inhale slowly and on the left side, *slowly* stretch the trunk upward and gradually curve it sideways toward the right.

   Begin from the left waistline to stretch the trunk upward and over, spreading the ribs apart, one from the other. The spine will curve to the right.

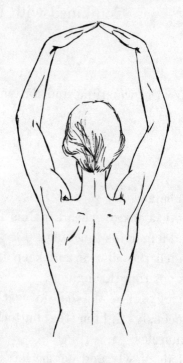

Arms overhead, fingers touching

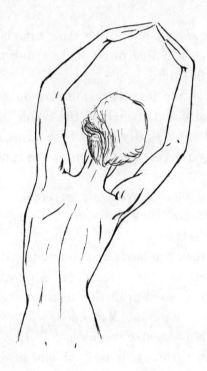

Bend sideways

Be careful to keep the body weight evenly distributed on both legs.

Bend sideways only as far as you can without causing a kink over the right waistline.

5. Exhale and hold the trunk in the side bend position.

6. Inhale *slowly*, and at the same time begin from the left waistline to raise the trunk to the upright position.

Use the long back muscles on the left to raise and straighten the trunk.

7. Exhale and slowly lower both arms sideways.

8. Slowly release the tension of the muscles just used.

9. Repeat these movements, stretching the right side of the trunk this time, bending the trunk to the left.

Because they are basic and complete with breathing instructions the preceding four Movement Schemes can be used profitably as a "daily review." Once familiar with the Mensendieck System, these Combined Movement Schemes can help you retain the vigor and grace your body should have.